AF659371

AIDS and Home Care

INTERNATIONAL ENCYCLOPAEDIA OF

AIDS

6

AIDS and Home Care

Editor
Dr. Digumarti Bhaskara Rao,
M.Sc., M.A., M.A., M.Ed., Ph.D.
R. V. R. College of Education
Guntur–522 006
Andhra Pradesh. (INDIA)

2000
DISCOVERY PUBLISHING HOUSE
NEW DELHI-110 002

First Published-2000

ISBN 81-7141-465-6 (Set)

© Editor

Published by:
DISCOVERY PUBLISHING HOUSE
4831/24, Ansari Road, Prahlad Street,
Darya Ganj, New Delhi-110 002 (*INDIA)*
Phone: 3279245
Fax: 91-11-3253475

Printed at:
Arora Offset Press
Laxmi Nagar, Delhi 110 092.

Preface

The HIV/AIDS is a new phenomenon in the human society. HIV destroys the immune system of human individuals, producing a defenselessness fatal state known as AIDS. The World Health Organisation has estimated that already one in every two hundred and fifty adults in the world is infected with Human Immunodeficiency Virus and according to WHO's projections a total of forty million men women and children worldwide will have been infected with HIV by the turn of this twentieth century. Visualising the devastating effects of the HIV/AIDS epidemic within our life times and beyond is difficult. Probably, no other disease in recent times has had the impact on human society generated by HIV/AIDS.

The HIV/AIDS epidemic has brought into focus many health related ethical, legal and human rights issues. This epidemic requires immediate and effective responses in new programming areas: attitudinal and behavioural changes, community-based care and support initiatives, and the maintenance of human development in the face of increasing rates of illness and deaths. At this point, education enters the scene as it can alter the HIV/AIDS situation since it brings change in the behaviour of the people.

This *International Encyclopaedia of AIDS* presents the worldwide information about HIV/AIDS, issues and challenges, reports and reviews, ethics laws and human rights, and educational activities and programmes to keep the policy makers, planners, professionals, activists, researchers, educationists, teachers and students well informed of the epidemic.

Dr. Digumarti Bhaskara Rao
26 January 1999
The Republic Day of India

Acknowledgement

I am thankful to the World Health Organisation and its associated offices for using their material namely School Health Education to prevent AIDS and STD: A Resource Package for Curriculum Planners-Handbook for Curriculum Planners. Student's Activities, Teachers' Guide, Global Programme on AIDS-HIV Prevention and Care: Teaching Modules for Nurses and Midwives, Global Programme on AIDS. Community HIV Prevention Handbook; STD care Management-workbooks 1-7, Facing the Challenge of HIV/ AIDS STDs: A Gender-based Response; HIV/AIDS and STD surveillance Data Management and Use-Report, Bangkok, 1995; Carrying out HIV Sentinal Surveillance-A Guide for Programme Managers, AIDS Prevention and Care in the workplace: Enhancing the Role of Private Sector; HIV Testing Policies and Guidelines; Carrying out HIV Sentinel surveillance; AIDS Prevention; Understanding and Living with AIDS; AIDS: A Modern Epidemic; HIV/AIDS in South-East Asia: IXth meeting of the National Programme Managers, New Delhi, 1993; Information, Education and Communication: A Guide for AIDS Programme Managers, Handbook on AIDS Home Care; HIV/AIDS in South-East Asia: A Pictorial summary; etc.

I am thankful to the United Nations Development Programme, UNDP's HIV and Development Programme, and UNDP's Regional Projects on HIV and Development for using their material namely Economic Implications of AIDS in Asia; Socio Economic Implications of the Epidemic; NGOs Working with Sex workers; NGO Responses to HIV/AIDS in Asia-Case Studies; HIV in the Workplace: Dealing with the Issues-Role Plays, Development and the HIV Epidemic, Law Ethics and HIV; HIV Law and Law Reform; Issue Papers; Study Papers; Working Papers; etc.

I am thankful to the Health and Nutrition Centre, Republic of Philippines for using its material namely sourcebook on HIV/AIDS Prevention Education for Tertiary Educational Institutions.

I am thankful to the Curriculum Development Programme, Ministry of Education, Government of Thailand for using its material namely Institutional Modules for AIDS Education.

I am thankful to US Department of Health and Human Services: Whitman-Walker Clinic, Inc., USA; East-West Centre, USA; National AIDS Control Organisation, Government of India; Academy of Culture Communication Education Science and Service, Guntur, United Nations and its agencies for using their material.

I am grateful to Bhaskar Bhattacharji; V. Alexeev, Geeta Sethi, Elizabeth Reid, Mina Mauerstein-Bail, A. A. Trinidad, Palomi Cuchi, D. Pushpa Latha for their kind co-operation.

Dr. Digumarti Bhaskara Rao,
Secretary
ACCESS
D-43, S.V. N. Colony,
Guntur-522 006

Contents

1

Teaching People with AIDS and Their Families

THE CARE you provide to people with HIV infection or AIDS may improve the quality and length of life, and help prevent the spreael of HIV and other associated illnesses. You may provide care in a hospital, clinic, home or any other location. In every place, teaching, i.e., sharing information and skills, is one of the most important tasks for a health care provider. Look at the pictures below:

- **Which of the following pictures shows a health care worker at work?**

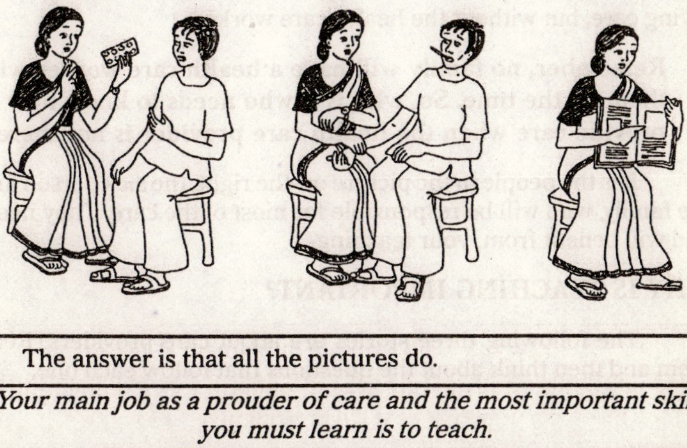

The answer is that all the pictures do.

Your main job as a prouder of care and the most important skill you must learn is to teach.

It will be difficult for you to take care of all the illnesses associated with HIV infection and AIDS and, with increasing numbers of people with HIV infection and AIDS, it is going to be even more difficult. Therefore, teaching becomes a crucial factor in providing care. One of the ways to help people with AIDS live positively is to make such people and their families capable of self-care.

WHOM SHOULD YOU TEACH?

As a provider of care, you are part of a group of people who work together to care for sick people, to maintain the health of people with HIV infection and to prevent the sprcad of HIV. List all care providers you can think of.

- **Did you remember to count the family members? ... the person with AIDS? ... and the members of the community?**

Look at the two pictures below:

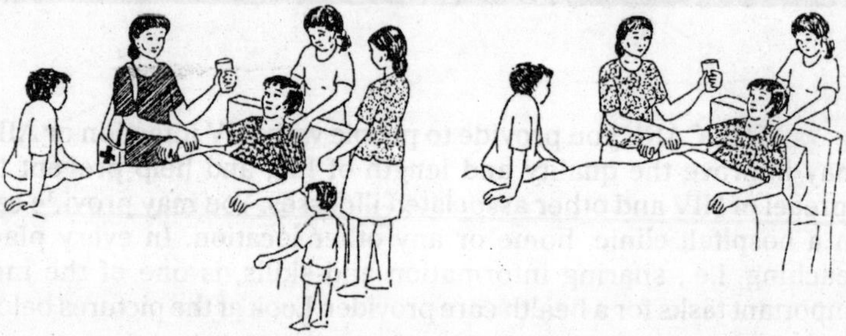

The picture on the left shows a family together with a health care worker caring for a sick person in a hospital, clinic or possibly in their home. The picture on thc right shows the same family, again giving care, but without the health care worker.

- **Remember, no family will have a health care worker with them all the time. So, who is it who needs to know how to provide care when the health care provider is not there?**

It is the people in thc picture on-the right, the sick person and the family, who will be responsible for most of the care. They need, and will benefit from, your teaching.

WHY IS TEACHING IMPORTANT?

The following three stories are about care providers. Read them and then think about the questions that follow each one.

STORY A

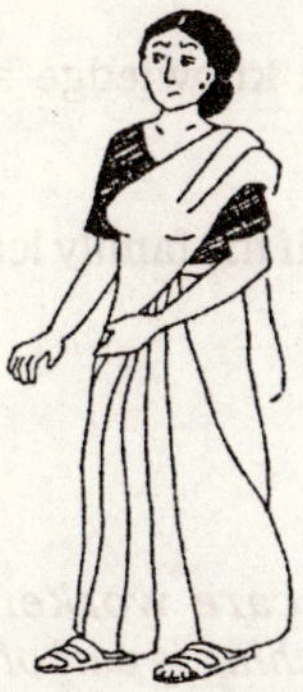

Mrs. Kamini a health care worker in India, visits the home of Ramu who has AIDS and is suffering from cough. She carries out all her tasks just the way she has been trained. She is very efficient. She tells the family she will come again the following week.

Mrs. Kamini comes back the following week, as she promised, but Ramu's cough has become worse. The family is upset and feel helpless.

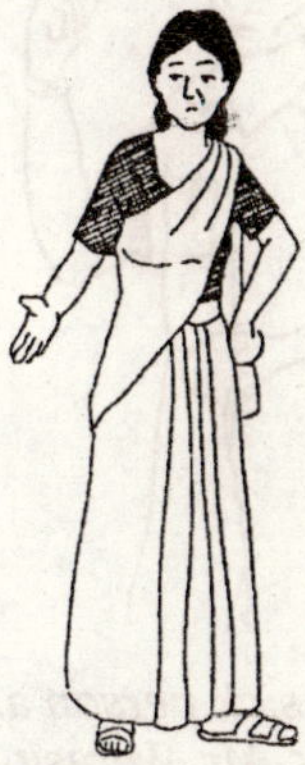

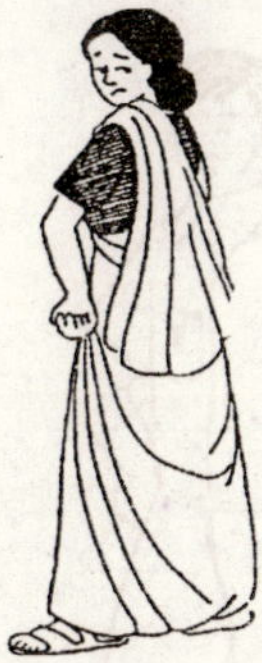

Mrs. Kamini continues to work efficiently but the situation does not improve much and, after a while, she starts to dislike visiting this family because it seems they are always complaining.

- **What has happened?**

Mrs. Kamini is kind to the family but she doesn't try to teach them any of the things she knows. While the family will certainly benefit from her visits, care will probably not help them become stronger in dealing with their problems. All of her useful knowledge goes away with her.

- **What are the reasons for this?**

Maybe ...

- Mrs. Kamini does not see the family as important members of the home care team
- she doesn't know or believe it is important to teach

- she doesn't know or believe families are able to take care of people with AIIDS
- she doesn't feel confident about her own knowledge and skills
- she doesn't know how or what to teach
- she thinks her importance will be lessened if the family learn what she knows

Do you have any other ideas?

STORY B

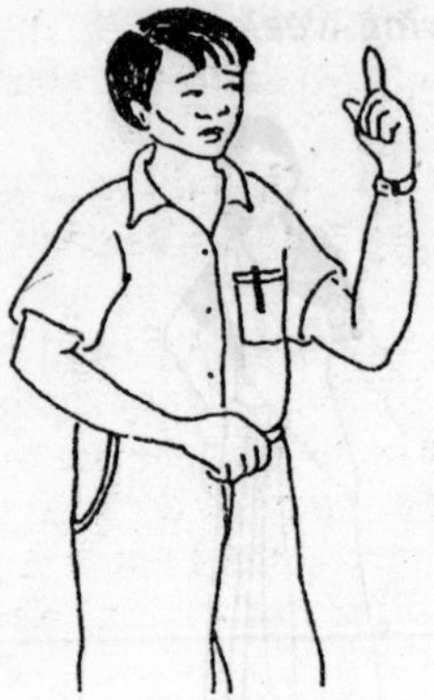

Mr. Werasit, a health care worker in Thailand, knows that teaching is part of his job. When the family of a person with AIDS comes to the clinic he tells them many facts while he carries out his duties. He tells them that diarrhoea is a common problem in AIDS and tells them how to prepare oral rebydration solution (ORS).

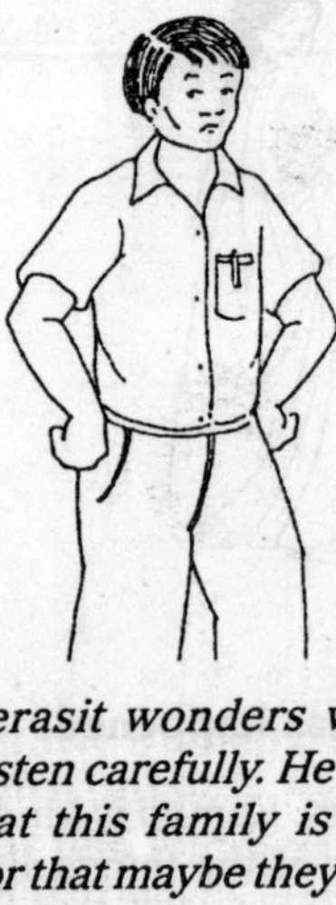

When the sick person and family come back, Mr. Werasit finds that they are not doing things the way he told them. He feels they can't even correctly remember much of the information on ORS which he gave during their previous visit.

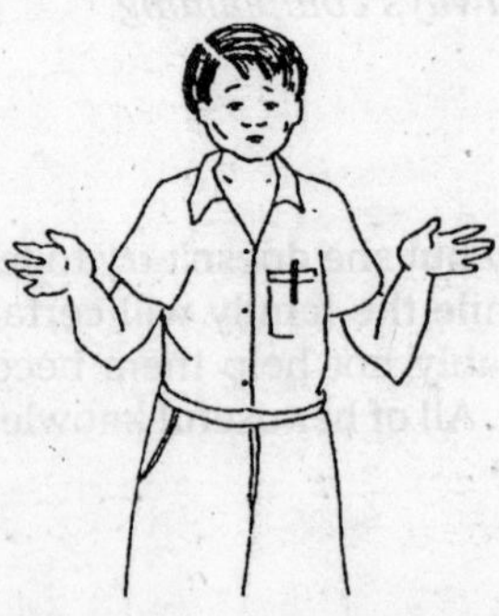

Mr. Werasit wonders why they don't listen carefully. He begins to feel that this family is not very smart or that maybe they just don't really care.

• WHAT HAS HAPPENED?

Mr. Werasit recognizes that families have a role in providing care. He thinks teaching is important, but he teaches the same way he was taught in school: he talks and they are supposed to listen. He gives them the advice and information, he feels, are important.

• WHY DIDN'T THIS WORK?

Maybe . . ..

- Mr. Werasit didn't tell them the information in a way they could understand
- he did not demonstrate the skills required for preparing ORS
- he didn't check if they understood what he had told them, or if they were able to carry out the directions he gave them
- he didn't give them a chance to ask questions and clarify doubts
- he didn't give them information that they believed was useful or important, that is, information they felt they needed to help them solve their problems.
- they already believed something completely different for example that the stomach should be kept empty during diarrhoea and therefore, had trouble believing what he said
- they didn't really have a chance to learn how to do what he taught; telling people how to do something does not ensure that they will have the skills, or will remember the steps, needed to do it.
- they didn't have the resources to do what he told them.
- Do you have any other ideas?

STORY C

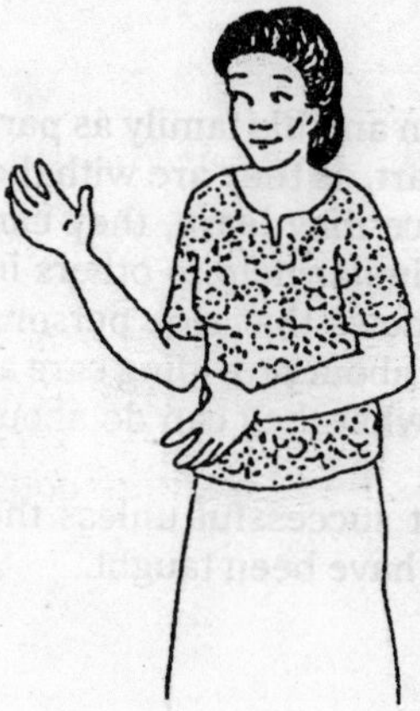

Mrs. Daw Kyi Kyi a health care worker in Myanmar, has taken care of Mr. U Than Tun since he was admitted in the hospital with high fever. Mr. U Than Tun has AIDS and is now getting ready to go home. His family has come to fetch him. Mr. U Than Tun and his family are a little afraid because at home there will be no medical care. Mrs. Daw Kyi Kyi understands their situation. She discusses their problems with Mr. U Than Tun and his family. She asks them which are the most troublesome problems for them. The family mentions fever as one of the problems. She listens to them carefully, discusses what to do at home and teaches them how to take care of somebody with fever at home.

She watches the family while they practise taking care of a person with fever. She tells them what problems to watch for and how to know they need to seek more help. Then she does some additional tasks, explaining her activities as she does them. She helps the family to think of other people in their community who might be able to give them assistance.

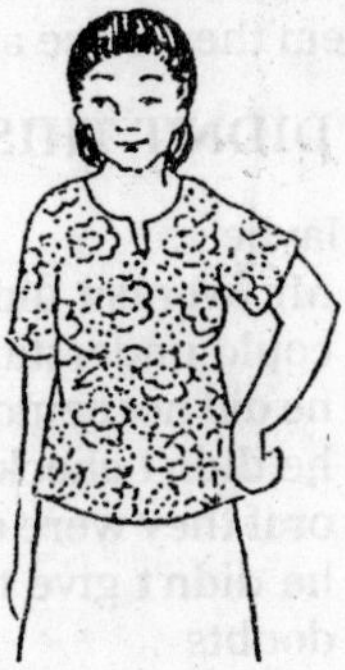

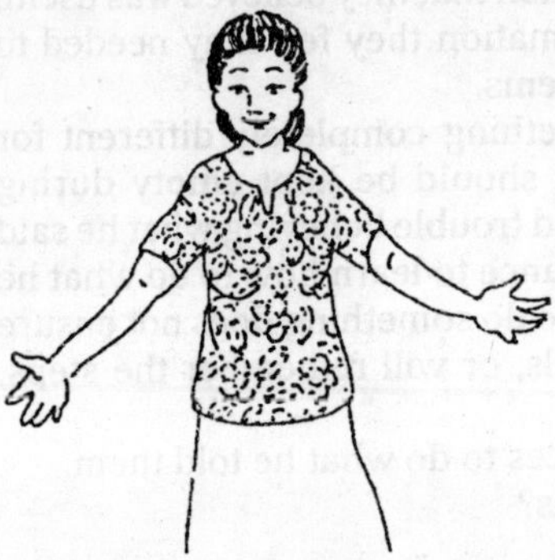

After one month, Mr. U Than Tun and his family come back to the hospital for a check-up. They ask to see Mrs. Daw Kyi Kyi. The family tell her they are feeling more comfortable and a little more capable of dealing with their problems. Mrs. U Than Tun says she has even been able to help a neighbour with a similar problem. They tell Mrs. Daw Kyi Kyi what else they feel they need to learn.

• What has happened?

Mrs. Daw Kyi Kyi sees Mr. U Than Tun and his family as part of the health care team - a very important part, as they are with the patient 24 hours a day. She knows that once they learn, they can provide the necessary care and also offer similar help to others in their community. Mrs. Daw Kyi Kyi also knows that sick persons and their family can become more confident about providing care at home if they know what is happening and what they can do about problems that arise.

She also knows that teaching is not successful unless the family has learned and practised what they have been taught.

• What did Mrs. Daw Kyi Kyi do?

- Mrs. Daw Kyi Kyi spent some of the time before Mr. U Than Tun left hospital giving and explaining the new information to the family - things they may not have known are important - and some of the time listening, and helping them with their own concerns.

- She taught them new skills (for example, cold sponging) step by step and helped them practise while she watched.
- She asked them questions and listened carefully to their answers because she wanted to know what, and how much, they understood.
- She also asked questions and listened to make sure that she correctly understood their concerns.
- She behaved in a way that made the family feel that she cared about them.

Mrs.. Daw Kyi Kyi was successful because she cared, and shared information.

Do you have any other ideas?

WHAT ARE THE BENEFITS OF TEACHING?

HIV infection and AIDS are often associated with a high level of stigma, fear and lack of acceptance of those affilicted. These feelings make it difficult to teach families about providing care at home, but through sharing information and skills, fear and stigma will decrease.

- People will learn the correct facts that they need to know and this will help tnem to accept people infected with HIV and people with AIDS.
- Thev will be less afraid to take care of people infected with HIV and will overcome part of the stigmatization and discrimination against those infected with HIV.
- People will learn to do things which will help them to stay healthy.
- They will know how to idcntify and manage common AIDS-related health problems in their homes.
- People will learn to recognise danger signs, and learn when and how to seek more help.
- They will feel more confident and comfortable because they are better able to help themselves and their family members.
- As a result of all of the above, sick people will receive better care and the load on the health care system will be decreased.

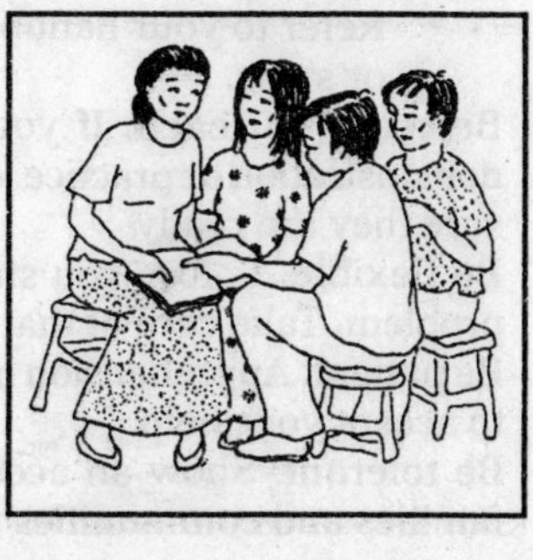

WHAT IS TEACHING?

Teaching is:

- Asking questions ... and listening
- Giving information ... and discussing information
- Checking to see whether

information is understood and accepted ... and asking questions
- Listening... and answering questions
- Showing people how to do a task correctly ... and helping them practise doing the task correctly
- Solving problems ... and helping people discover their own solutions to problems
- Listening... and asking questions
- Listening...

- **Why do you think "asking questions" and "listening" are repeated?**

Because these are the most important skills you can use to commulicate effectively with others and to teach them.

HOW SHOULD YOU TEACH?

- **Plan your teaching.**

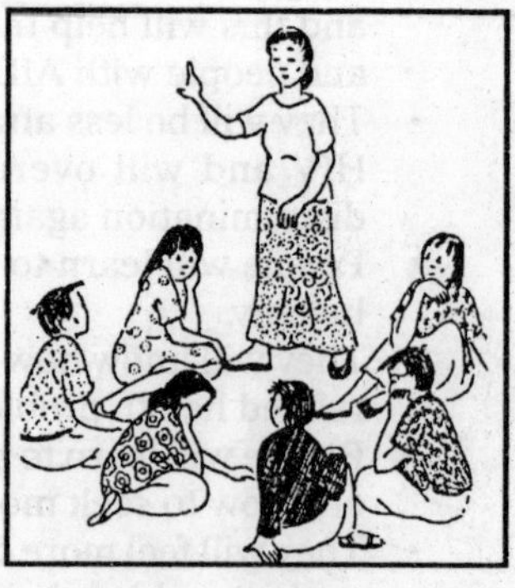

Decide what you will teach. What you teach should depend on what the sick person and his or her family want and need to know at different times. Build on what they already know.
- You may find that making and using a checklist of priority topics for teaching is helpful.

Make sure your information is correct. Preparing your information ahead of time will help you to make sure of this.
- Use this handbook to prepare and check your information.

Be organized. Plan what you will say. Make sure you can remember all the steps of a procedure or treatment.
- Refer to your handbook, or make a list of important points or steps.

Be ready to teach. If you have or need special materials for demonstration or practice, or pictures to help explain points, make sure they are ready.

Be flexible. Before you start, find out if there is a more urgent problem. Take care of that first.

Be patient. Apprehension in families can make it difficult for them to accept your help.

Be tolerant. Show an accepting, caring attitude. This will help families and communities to become more accepting too.

Be prepared. React quickly to your audience, and adapt your teaching if necessary as you go along.
Plan for a review to see whether the person/family has understood and can perform the tasks you had taught them.
Use as far as possible the family's own language.

- **Help those you teach feel comfortable.**

Be sympathetic and understanding.
Treat them as equals.
Talk politely to them.
Use words they can understand.
Respect their beliefs and traditions.
Respect their independence.
Avoid being judgemental.
Encourage them to ask questions and talk, and remember:

- listen to them carefully
- show respect for what they say
- show an accepting, caring attitude. This will help families and communities become more accepting too.

- **Keep your teaching simple: too much information all at once is confusing.**
- **Make sure you find out what the family and the sick person know or believe.**

Ask questions:

- to find out what they already know, believe, or plan to do about their problems
- to find out whether you understand correctly what their concerns are
- to make sure they understand correctly what you have told them
- to make sure they are satisfied with the answers they have received
- to find out what else they might need to know
- to learn from them.
- Make sure you demonstrate how to provide care.
- Ask them to demonstrate to you after you show them how.

When you are asked something that you don't know, say ...
"I don't know but I will find out for you.".

- **What is wrong with this answer?**

Nothing. If you aren't sure of something, the best thing to do is to say so. Tell the family you will find out the answer to their question. Make sure you do find out and tell them as soon as you can. In this way you have shown respect for their question and they will not lose confidence or respect for you.

WHAT SHOULD YOU TEACH?

First, remember:

The sick person and the family have the main responsibility for giving care at home. They must also be able to protect and promote their own and each other's health.

Ask yourself: "What do they need to know in order to do this?

Focus oll teaching the skills and knowledge that will be useful and valuable to them.

They need to know all of the following things:

- what HIV anc' AIDS are
- how HIV is transmitted (and how it is not transmitted)
- how to find out if a person is infected with HIV
- what problems or symptoms are commonly associated with AIDS
- how to recognize and take care of common emotional and physical problems caused by HIV infection and AIDS
- when it is important to seek additional help and where to go for this
- where to go for counselling
- how to lead as normal and satisfying a life as possible
- what they can do to prevent the transmission of HIV
- that there may be stigma associated with HIV infection and AIDS
- what common myths are associated with HIV infection and AIDS
- what their legal and human rights are
- how to protect care givers from infection
- that care givers themselves have emotional needs.

- **How can you help the people you know and work with to be sure they have guidance on all these points?**

Immediately after a person has learnt that they have HIV infection or AIDS, they and their family will probably want to know exactly what AIDS is and how to prevent HIV transmission in the home. They will need help in dealing with the emotional shock of the diagnosis. They will also need to know that there is much they can all do to protect their own health.

As the disease progresses and people have had time to understand and accept the situation, they will probably become more interested in the specific physical anel emotional symptoms which they experience.

Later, as the sick person moves into the chronic and finally the terminal stages of AIDS, they may become more interested in practical concerns such as making preparations for the care of children, or the settling of finances, as well as in the spiritual and emotional preparation for dying.

This is only a general pattern. Each sick person and each family remains unique.

The information in this handbocak, if carefully explained, should not be too difficult for anyone to understand.

HERE ARE SOME MORE STORIES ABOUT TEACHING:

STORY D

Mrs. Thapa from Kathmandu was very worried her grandchildren would get AIDS from their mother, who had recently become sick. It was all she could think about on Wednesday when Mrs. Bhandari, the health care worker, visited them at home. Before Mrs. Thapa could tell her fears, Mrs. Bhandari sat down with her and began teaching her about the importance of nutrition for people with AIDS. She gave Mrs. Thapa lots of good advice and information. Mrs. Thapa hardly heard a word, her mind was so full of worries about her grandchildren. Without bothering to find out whether Mrs. Thapa had any questions, Mrs. Bhandari moved on to the next family.

Mrs. Bhandari gave her correct and useful information and spoke politely and clearly, but afterwards Mrs. Thapa couldn't remember what she had told her.

- **Why didn't Mrs. Thapa learn?**

Maybe . ..

Mrs. Bhandari gave the correct information, but at the wrong time. She didn't find out what things were worrying Mrs. Thapa most and address those things first. If she had, then Mrs. Thapa would have been reassured and could have concentrated on what Mrs. Bhandari was telling her about nutrition.

STORY E

Mrs. Saheda from Bangladesh is a health care worker. She had come first in her training group and was proud of her training. She knew many medical words now, and how to use them correctly. But many of thefamilies she dealt with were uneducated. She tried to teach them, but they didn't seem to learn. They didn't even ask questions.

- **What do you think was happening?**

Maybe ...

Mrs. Saheda forgot that talking at someone isn't the same as teaching them. Teaching means making sure the learner has understood and is able to use what has been taught. People need to feel comfortable in order to learn. Mrs. Saheda needed to use words that a sick person and his or her family could easily understand.

YOU CAN TEACH!

Teaching can take place anywhere. You can teach in the hospital, the outpatient clinic or in someone's home. You might be able to think of other places where informal teaching can take place. Teaching should be done during every contact with the person or the family. You have valuable information. Sharing it may save someone's life.

In order to make this handbook more useful to you, space has been provided at the end of each health problem section in Chapter Six for your own notes. As you learn about ways or methods that help the people you work with .n your community, write them in. Often the best solutions to problems are the ones people discover for themselves.

Caring and sharing information will help people with HIV infection or AIDS their families to live positively.

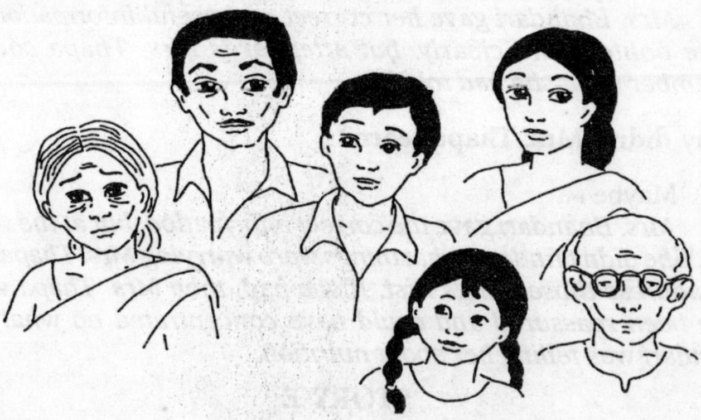

2

From HIV Infection to AIDS

Prevention of transmission of HIV, which causes AIDS, is the most important strategy to reduce the impact of the epidemic. Knowledge about HIV and AIDS and how HIV is transmitted and not transmitted is very important in preventing the spread of the epidemic, and also in helping those affected by HIV and AIDS to live positively and to care for themselves.

Most people find that information about HIV transmission and AIDS is very difficult to teach to others. The details are hard grasp even for scientists, so it is no wonder that people in the community have problems understanding the important points and acting on this information in ways that are helpful.

A story can be a very useful and effective way of explaining the key issues surrounding HIV and AIDS. This handbook tells two stories the first onc is about the impact of AIDS on a family, and the second about a young man who is infected with HIV through injecting drugs. The stories are told first. This is followed by—teaching notes that look at the stories in detail, explaining what has happened and providing more information about HIV and AIDS. The information is presented in a way that you can use directly when teaching.

The first story continues through Chapters 3 and 4 and ends in Chaptcr 5.

Here are some suggestions for using the stories:

- Tell the stories (or your own variation of them) and then go through them again slowly, asking questions and providing information. You can tell a story in many parts, as suggested here, examining each part in detail before you go on, or you might prefer to tell the whole story right through first. You can keep coming back to the stories in your teaching sessions, reminding your audience of what happened to the family and the young man this will help you to explain the different issues involved.

- Full-page versions of some of the pictures used here are provided at the back of this book. You might find these larger pictures useful when telling a story.
- Be sure that you change the stories to make them familiar to the people you are talking to. For example, change the names to ones that are common in your area. If you are telling the stories in a rural setting you could say that the people are from the village where you are and then describe a journey to a city that is familiar to everyone in the village. You want the people hearing the stories to think "Yes, I know these people". However, be careful not to talk about anybody in particular.
- Review background information before telling the stories so that you are clear on the facts and prepared to answer questions as they arise.
- Make the level of information and the words you use suitable for the people hearing the stories and for what they already know. The questions given along the way in a story are a guide. However, encourage your listeners to ask their own questions too.
- live your audience time to answer questions and tell you what is happening, before explaining things clearly yourself.
- You can also tell these stories with the pictures and make sure that the time at which the events occur is clear. To do this, you might first want to put the dates up on the wall, and as you tell the stories and show the pictures you can then place the pictures on the wall under the date on which the events described happen. Please note that you can change the dates in the stories to suit the date of storytelling.

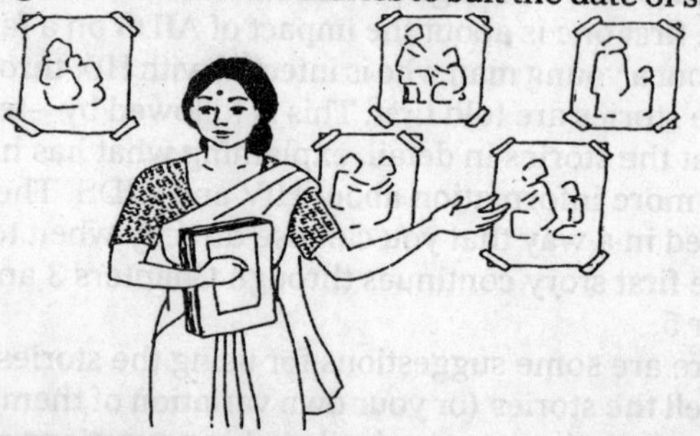

- Remember that using storytelling as a teaching method means that the stories should be made lively, the audience must be encouraged to think by asking questions.
- You are not trying to shock or scare people - only to provide them with useful and correct information.

- Talking to people about sexual matters has to be done sensitively. Do not feel embarrassed and if possible use terms that are seen as sensitive or polite by the community.

STORY I: RADHA AND RAVI

This story is used to show how HIV comes into a family and what happens over the years. The characters are shown in pictures to make it more interesting.

EARLY 1983

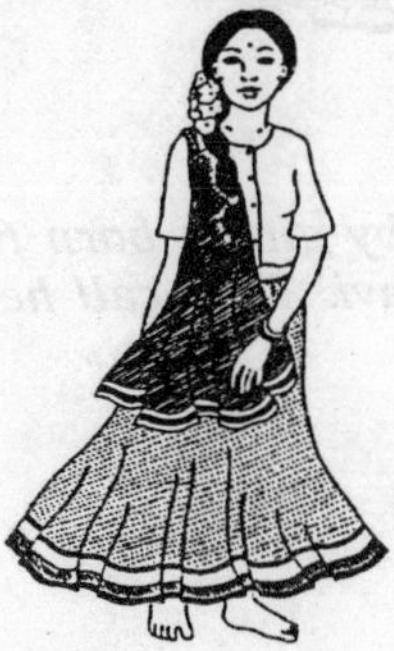

This is Radha, from a village in India She is a very intelligent girl and has done well in school. This is her last year in school. Radha's parents are proud of her and are very anxious to find her a good husband as she is already eighteen. They plan to arrange her marriage as soon as she finishes school. Radha's maternal uncle comes to visit them. Radha's parents request him to find a boy for Radha. A few week's later Radha's uncle brings a marriage proposal for Radha. The parents are pleased with the proposal—The marriage is fixed.

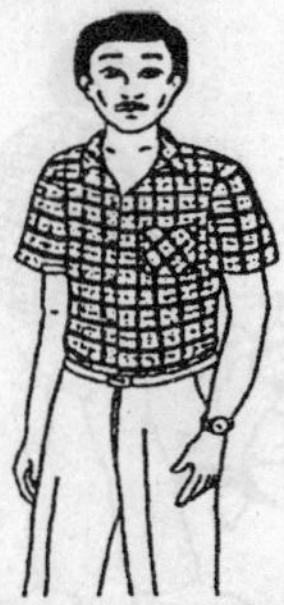

This is Ravi. Ravi works as a supervisor in a factory. He works hard. He is well-respected and liked by his colleagues and superiors. He is happily engaged to Radha.

LATE 1983

Ravi and Radha are married in the traditional Indian style. There is a big celebration, everyone comes.

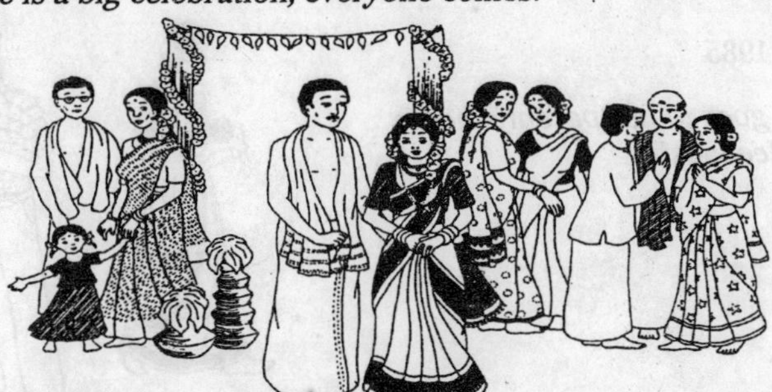

Radha and Ravi live together in the town where Ravi works.

MID-1984

Radha becomes pregnant. Both Radha and Ravi are happy. The families of both Radha and Ravi are also very excited.

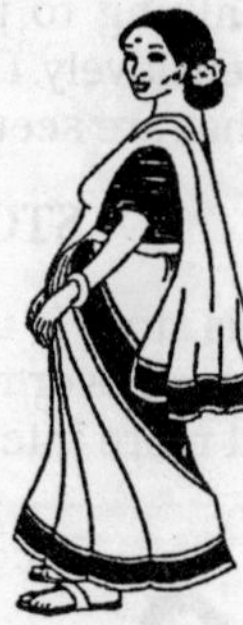

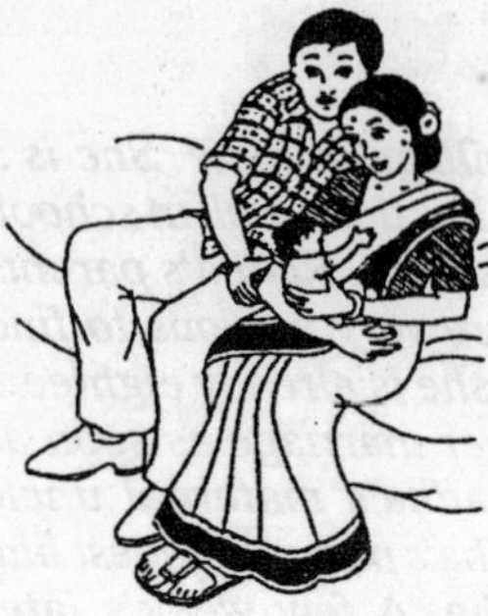

EARLY 1 985

A healthy baby girl is born to Radha and Ravi. They call her Meenakshi.

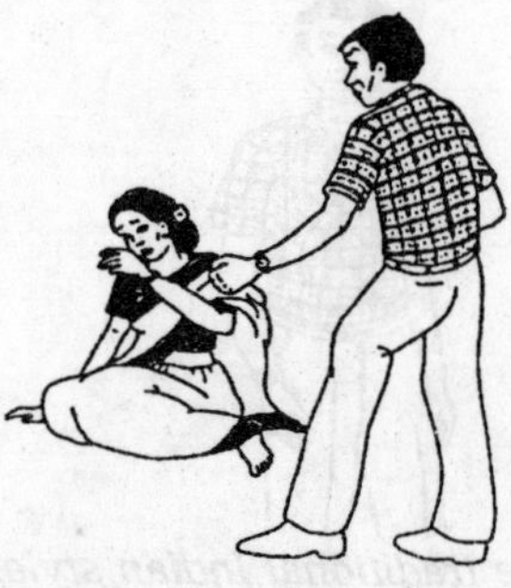

MID-1985

Srinivasan is a friend of Ravi. He is an alcoholic and Ravi starts drinking with him regularly. Ravi gets into a bad mood when he is drunk. He beats Radha at the slightest provocation. Radha is unhappy.

LATE 1985

Radha goes to her parent's home with Meenakshi.

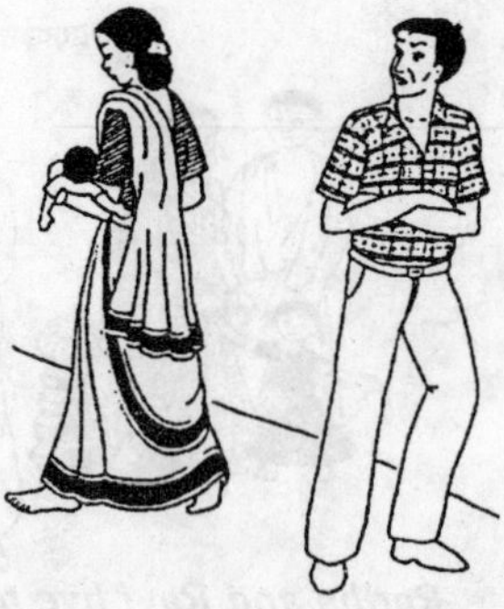

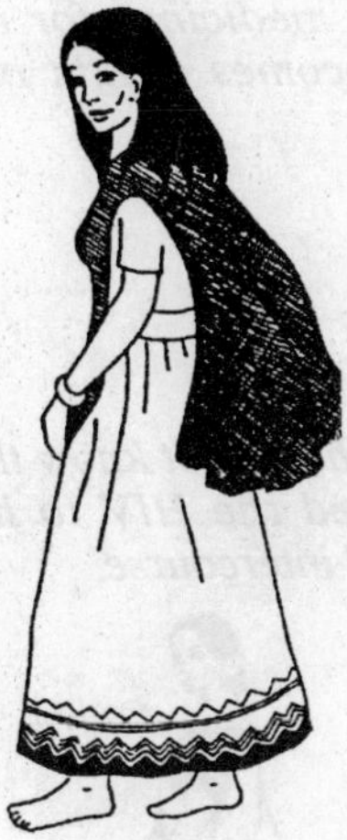

Ravi feels very upset and lonely. He misses Radha and Meenakshi. He spends more time in the company of Srinivasan. Srinivasan has several girl friends. He introduces Ravi to Remani and encourages him to befriend her. Ravi does not want to be unfaithful to Radha. So, be ignores Srinivasan's suggestions. One day, after drinking a lot of alcohol, Ravi goes to visit Remani. Ravi finds Remani's company interesting and his loneliness decreases. He also has sex with her without using a condom. A week or so later, Ravi notices some painful sores on his penis, which disappear after treatment. Even though the sexually transmitted disease (STD) is cured, the HIV, which was transmitted at the same time, remains in Ravi's body - unknown to him.

MID-1986

Ravi's brother finds out about his relationship with another woman and talks to him. Ravi promises his brother that he will not have sexual relationships with other women again. He also promises not to beat Radha again. Ravi goes to Radha's parents' home and apologizes to Radha. He brings Radha and Meenakshi back to their home. The family is happy to be together again.

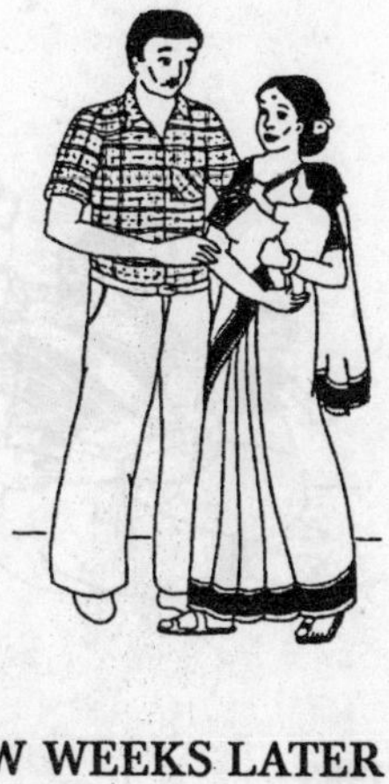

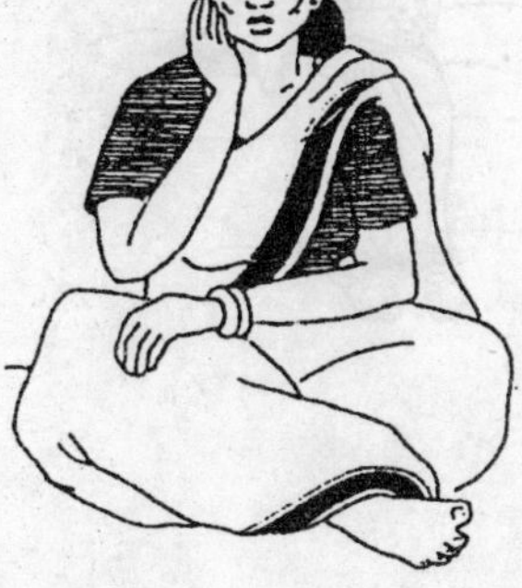

MID-1986 – A FEW WEEKS LATER

Radha and Ravi continue to have sexual intercourse. They do not use a condom.

Radha develops fever and has a few red spots on her body.

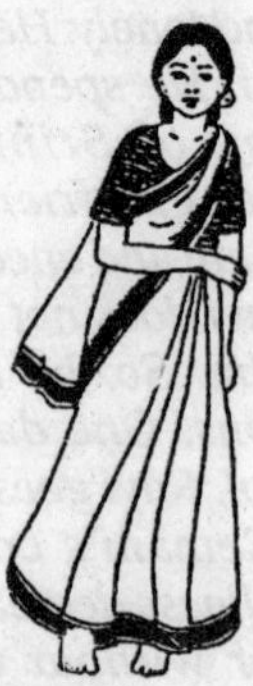

Radha takes medicines for the fever and becomes alright in a week's time.

Ravi and Radha do not know that he has passed the HIV to her during sexual intercourse.

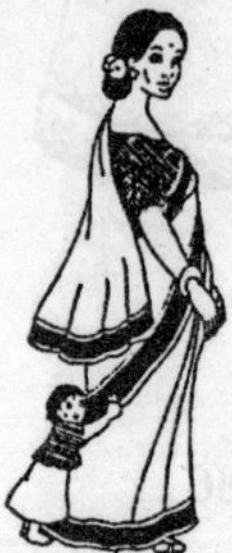

EARLY 1987

Life is good for Ravi and Radha. Ravi gets a promotion. Radha is pregnant again.

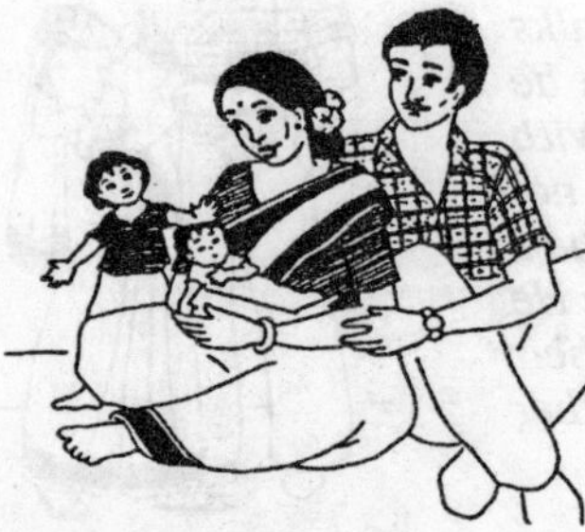

LATE 1987

Radha and Ravi are blessed with another child a boy named Kannan.

The new baby is infected with HIV.

1988

Kannan is on breast milk, but he gets frequent diarrhoea and fever. He is not gaining weight as he should. Radha is very worried. She visits many child specialists, but Kannan's situation deteriorates. Kannan is six months old now, but he weight only 3 kilograms.

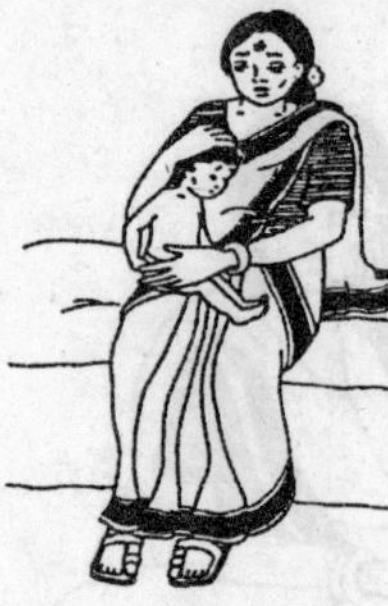

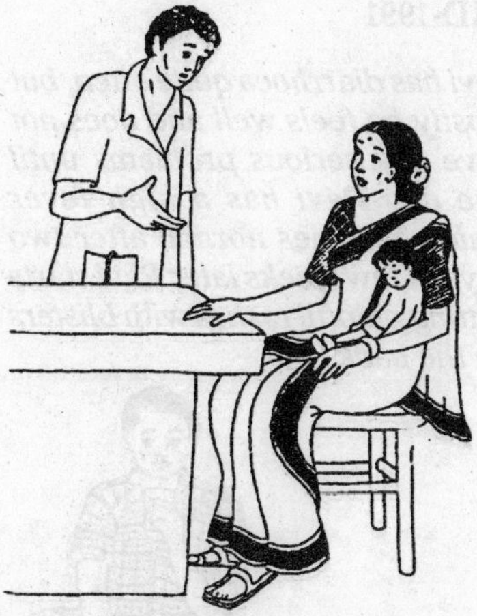

It is during one of her visits to the doctor that she is asked a few personal questions, some of which embarrass her. The doctor asks about her relationship with her husband and also whether her husband has been seeing other women. He explains to her why he is asking these questions and tells her about an illness called AIDS. The doctor tells Radha that the child may have AIDS. He says that he cannot tell from a blood test until the baby is fifteen months old. He talks to Radha about having a blood test, along with her husband. He spends time talking to her about the test. Radha is shocked to bear what the doctor says and does not believe that she or Ravi could have the infection. But she agrees to have the test done because the doctor is a kind man. Radha goes home, but never tells any of this to Ravi. She does not have the courage to ask Ravi whether he had relationships with other women. She never bothers to find out the results of her blood test.

LATE 1988

Kannan continues to fall sick. Radha goes to a traditional healer who gives her some powder and assures her that Kannan will recover. But, one morning when Radha wakes up, she finds that Kannan has died. The family is very sad. Luckily, for Radha and Ravi, Meenakshi remains healthy and is a comfort.

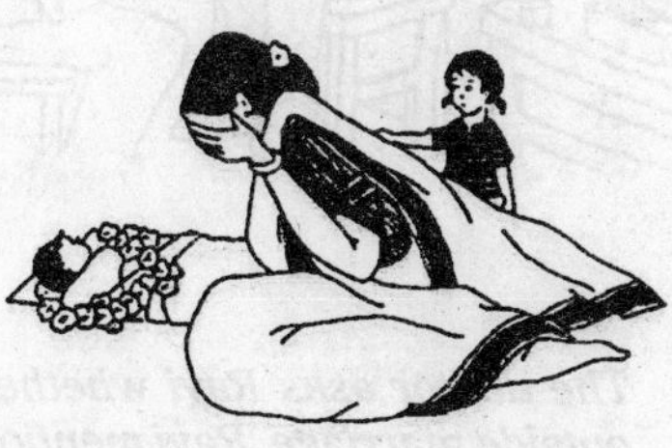

Slowly, Radha and Ravi get over the sorrow of losing Kannan. Sometimes Radha remembers what the doctor had told her and about her test. Still she doesn't bother to find out the result of the test or discuss it with Ravi.

MID-1991

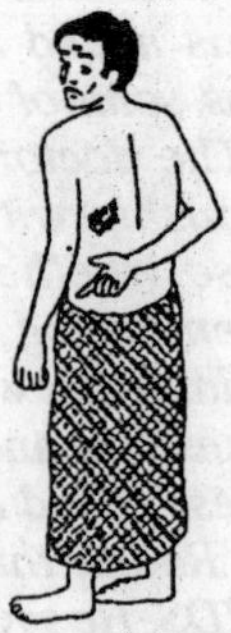

Ravi has diarrhoea quite often, but mostly he feels well and does not have any serious problems until one day Ravi has a high fever which becomes normal after two days. A few weeks later Ravi starts getting painful rashes with blisters on the back.

He becomes alright after a week.

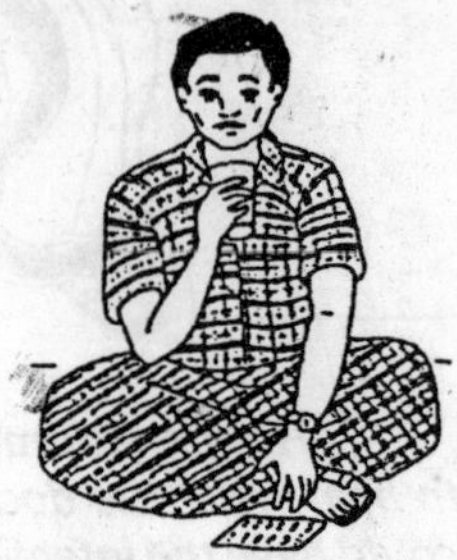

LATE 1991

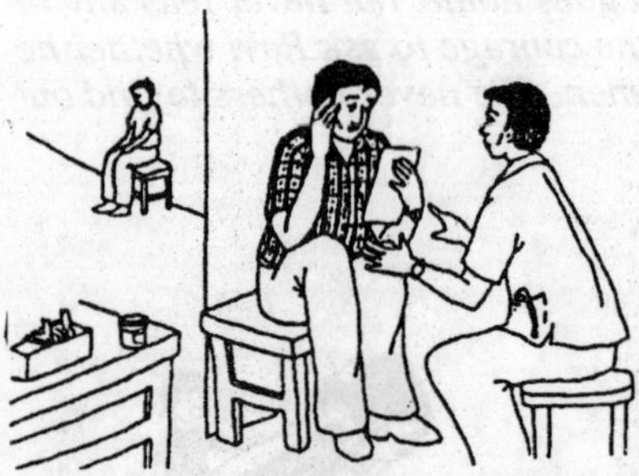

Ravi feels very tired and is losing weight. He often falls sick sometimes diarrhoea, sometimes fever. He consults a doctor who suspects that he may be developing AIDS.

The doctor asks Ravi whether he had any sexual relationships outside marriage. Ravi mentions his "visits" with another woman. The doctor tells him about HIV infection and asks Ravi to get a blood test done to see whether he has HIV. Ravi agrees.

A week later Ravi returns to the doctor and he is told that his test is positive. The doctor tells him what could happen to him and how he should take care of himself He also asks Ravi to get his wife tested as he may have infected her. Ravi tells the doctor about Kannan. The doctor tells Ravi that Kannan probably died of AIDS.

Ravi is totally devastated. He doesn't know how to face Radha He is very depressed and afraid of death. He is worried about Radha and Meenakshi. He feels responsible for Kannan's death. He never discusses his test results with Radha

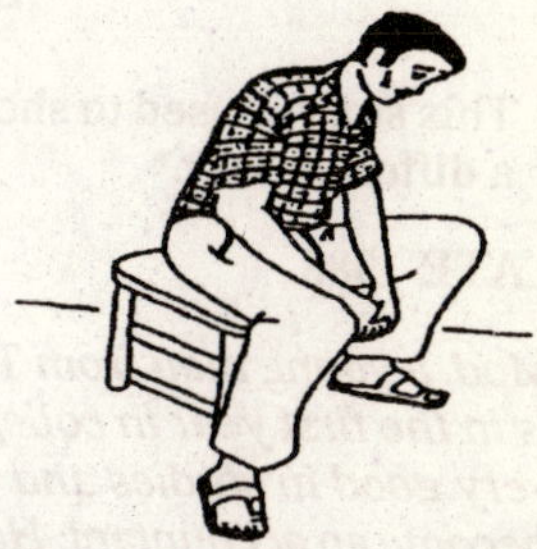

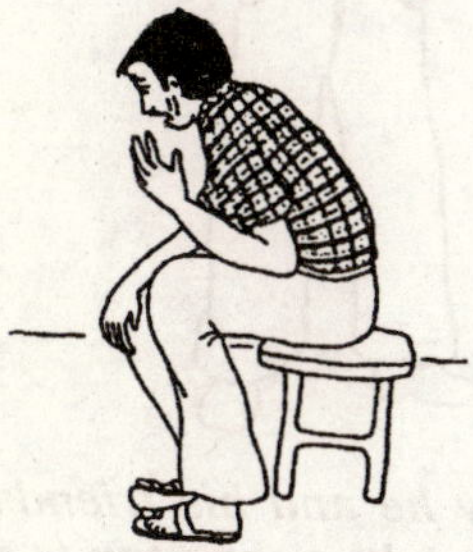

EARLY 1992

Ravi has been coughing for a few weeks and one evening, he coughs out blood from his mouth. Ravi is diagnosed as having tuberculosis and is put on treatment. Ravi does well on medicines and after six months he is told that he is cured of tuberculosis.

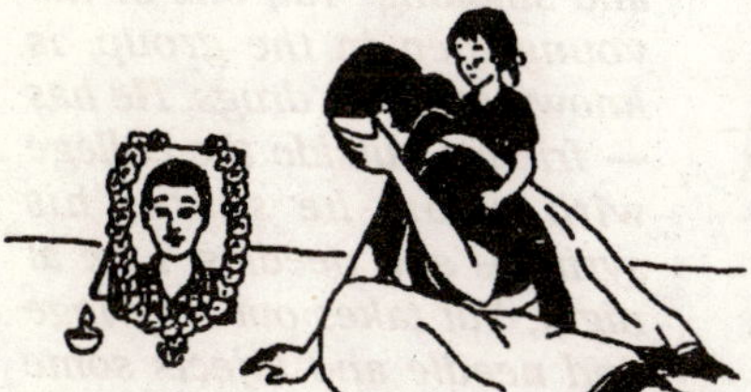

EARLY 1993

Ravi gets pneumonia He is admitted in the hospital Ravi feels very weak and finds it difficult to even sit up. He quits his Job. His condition deteriorates. He is in pain most of the time. He also becomes very irritable and is always getting annoyed with Radha and Meenakshi. One day Ravi dies and is cremated.

The months and years since Kannan's death and during Ravi's illness have been bad for Radha is physically and emotionally worn out caring for Ravi. She often remembers what Kannan's doctor said. She starts thinking that maybe both Kannan and Ravi died of the same illness. She wonders whether her test results came out positive. She is very anxious about Meenakshi's future. Her parents have been a great source of strength and support to her. She knows she can count on them.

During the months after Ravi's death, Radha slowly picks up courage and becomes emotionally strong.

Let us leave this story here for now and go to the second story.

STORY 2: MOD

This story is used to show bow a young man gets HIV infection in a different way.*

LATE 1988

Mod, a young man from Thailand, is in the first year in college. He is very good in studies and wants to become an accountant. He stays in the college hostel He notices some of his friends taking drugs. He is curious about these drugs as he has heard that they give a big 'kick, but he is not interested in trying them out.

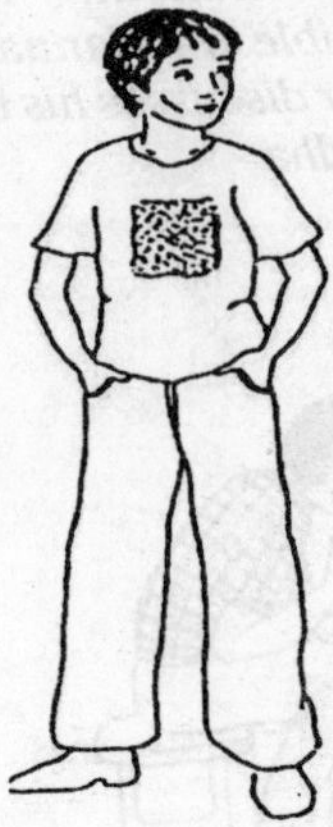

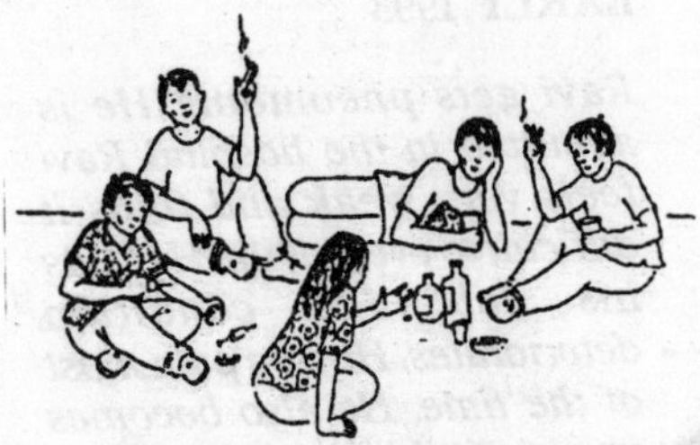

One day he and his friends decide to take a short trip to a beach which is close by. They have great fun drinking beer and smoking. Yut, one of the young men in the group, is known to inject drugs. He has — friends outside the college with whom he shares his syringes and needles. Late at night, Yut takes out a syringe and needle and injects some brown fluid. He encourages his friends also to do the same.

Mod is scared, but on his friend's insistence, he agrees to try the injection. They all share the same syringe and needle. Soon Mod feels as though he is flying. It is a fantastic feeling.

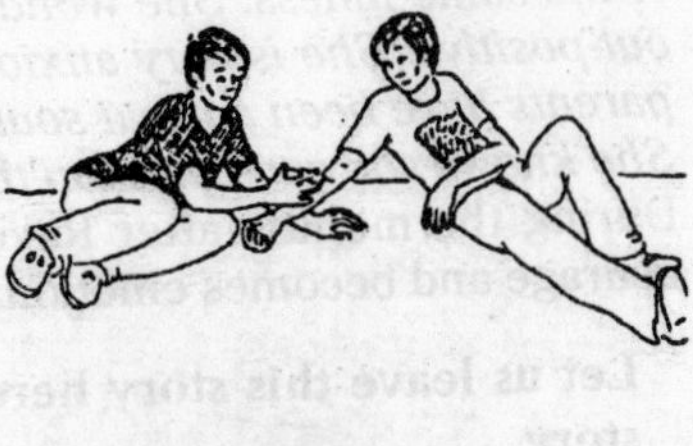

1989

Mod and his friends start using the drugs regularly in the hostel and they always inject drugs using the same needle and syringe. They never clean these syringes and needles. Mod gets addicted to drugs. He spends all the money which his parents send him to buy drugs and requests time and again for more money. Mod does not know that he has been infected with HIV while sharing a syringe and needle.

MID-1990

Mod loses interest in his studies and stops going to college. His parents are very concerned. Mod's mother sees him stealing money. She tells her husband about this. They watch Mod closely and suspect that he is on drugs. They also fear a new disease they have heard about that they know can be transmitted while injecting drugs using dirty needles.

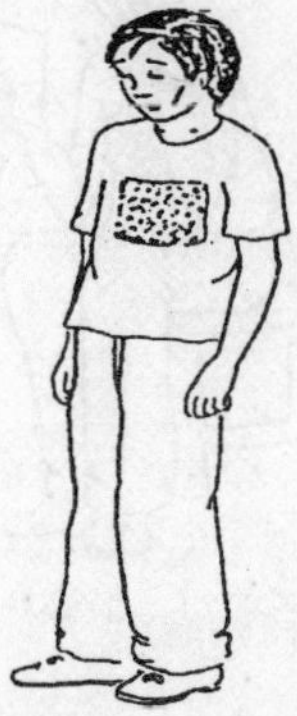

LATE 1991

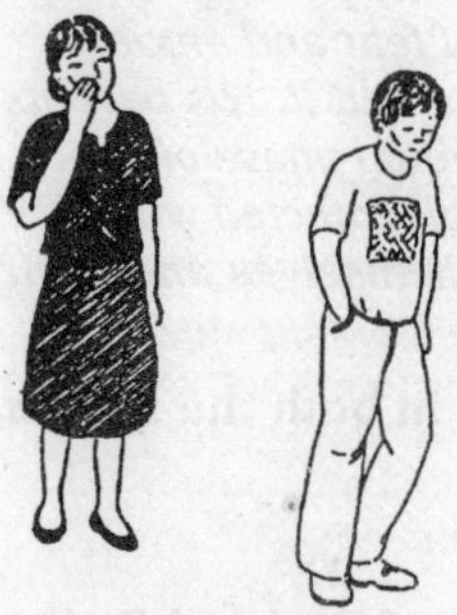

Mod steals money frequently. One day his mother sees him injecting drugs and she tells her husband. The parents are very scared, upset and angry with Mod. They try everything to get him out of the addiction, including warning him about a disease called AIDS. Finally, they get him admitted to a drug rehabilitation centre where he also hears more about the danger of sharing needles.

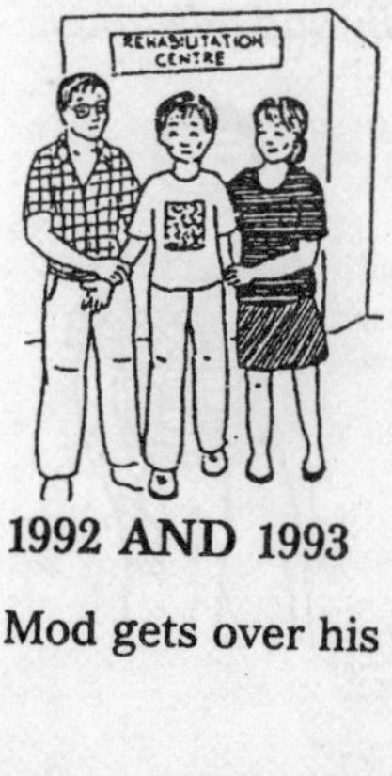

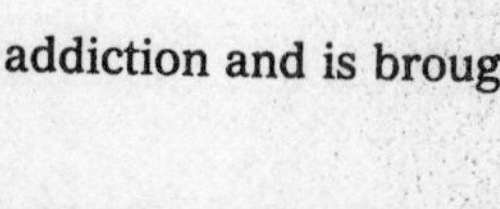

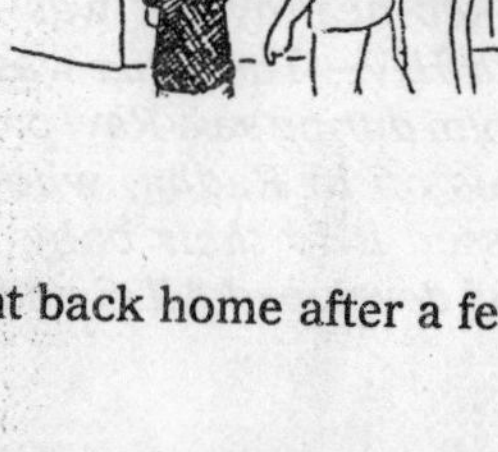

1992 AND 1993

Mod gets over his addiction and is brought back home after a few months. In spite of the warnings about HIV/AIDS, be starts injecting drugs again and his parents take him back to the rehabilitation centre. He gets over the addiction and is brought back home. Within a short time, he is tempted again and starts using drugs. But this time he decides to seek help himself: He goes back again to the rehabilitation centre.

1994

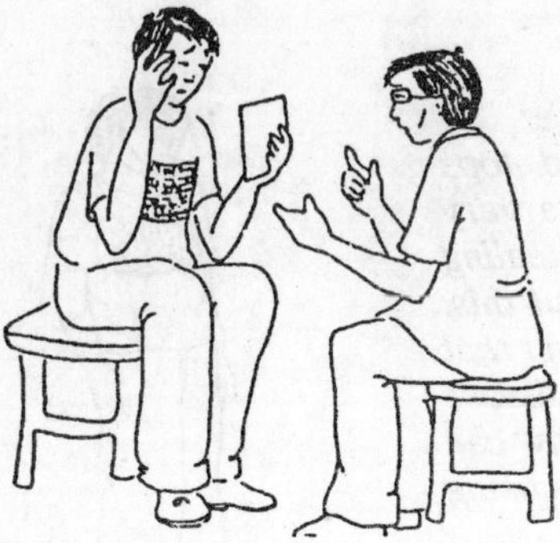

Mod has got over the addiction in the rehabilitation centre and stays "clear" with the ongoing help of a counsellor who talks with him regularly. It is almost six months since Mod has injected drugs. One day Mod shares his fears of AIDS with his counsellor who suggests that he should probably get himself tested for HIV He talks to him about the test. Mod's blood test shows that he has HIV infection. Mod is devastated. He wants to run away. The counsellor in the centre helps him through this period of fear and anxiety.

Mod picks up courage and tells his parents about it. His parents give him support and help him through the initial phase of shock. Mod is now actively working with other people infected with HIV and also educating drug users to protect themselves and their partners from this disease.

- **Let us think about what has happened in both the stories.**

TEACHING NOTES ON HIV AND AIDS

Take your audience back through the story of Ravi and Radha, following the course of the infection in this family and talk about what their story shows.

- **What has happened to the family?**

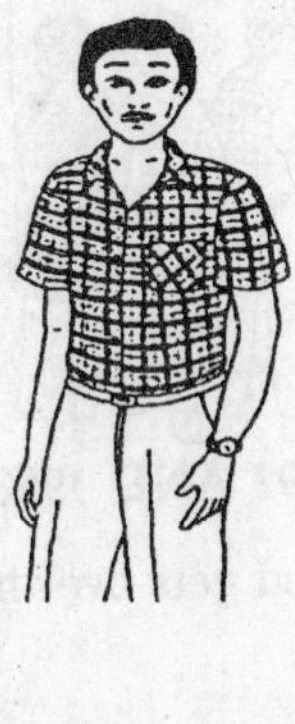

The story started when Ravi had unprotected sex with Remani who looked healthy but was infected with HIV~ The virus was passed to him during sex. Ravi passed the virus on to Radha, who in turn passed it to their baby Kannan. Ravi developed AIDS and died.

WHAT ARE HIV AND AIDS?

The disease AIDS the acquired immunodeficiency syndrome is caused by a virus, the human immunodeficiency virus (HIV). Viruses are very small organisms which cannot be seen by the naked eye. They cause many different diseases in humans and animals. Poliomyelitis (polio) is another example of a disease caused by a virus. Viruses cannot survive on their own and can multiply only in human or animal bodies.

HOV' DOES HIV AFFECT THE BODY'S IMMUNF SYSTEM?

- **The immune system**

White blood cells (WBCs) are a very important part of what is called the immune system. The immune system, with its WBCs, defends the body from infections. It recognizes bacteria, viruses and other organisms that are foreign or dangerous to the body and begins to attack them. It also starts making specific substances called antibodies which act against the particular disease-causing organism that has infected the body. White blood cells can be compared to soldiers in a country. The soldiers are always on the watch for enemics and the moment they sense enemy presence, they defend the country.

- **Weakening the immune system**

When a person becomes infected with HIV, the virus begins to live and reproduce in the WBCs, multiplying until there are millions of viruses present. The WBCs begin to make antibodies to HIV which are found in the blood about 6 to 12 weeks after infection. Unfortunately, these antibodies cannot eliminate the virus completely from the body as the virus is hides in the WBCs. The virus gradually damages the WBCs so that they can no longer do their job of protecting the body from other kinds of infections, which healthy people without HIV can normally fight off without any problem. It is when these infections occur that a person is said to have AIDS.

The bacteria, viruses and parasites present in the environment that cause these infections take the opportunity given by the weakened immune system to grow unhindered. This is why many of the illness that people with AIDS get are called opportunistic infections. Common conditions, such as tuberculosis or cancer, can also take advantage of the weakened immune system.

The above process is shown in the cartoon shown on next page:

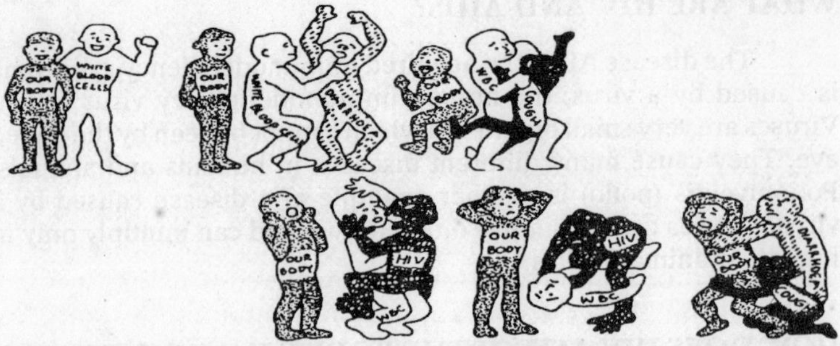

WHAT HAPPENS IN HIV INFECTION?

Ravi remained well for many years after he got infected. But as the virus started destroying more of the WBCs, he started feeling sick. Two years before he died, he developed fever and painful rashes on his body. He started losing weight. He also suffered from frequent illnesses after that. He was suffering from tuberculosis a year before his death, which was cured with treatment. Then he got pneumonia. His condition deteriorated and finally he died. Let us see what happened to Radha. Radha had a flu-like illness initially after which she remained well.

In the early stages of HIV infection (within weeks), the person may develop a flu-like illness with fever and may have rashes. The person gets well after a few days. But the person can already pass on the virus to another person. Not all infected people develop this kind of initial illness.

A person with HIV may look and feel healthy and may remain so for many years. It is not unusual for the period of time between infection with HIV and becoming ill with AIDS to be eight or nine years, and sometimes as long as 15 years. The length of time can vary widely in different people. But, the person can pass on the virus to another person even while he or she looks healthy.

After this time, people with HIV begin to feel sick with minor illnesses such as low grade fever, rashes, infections of the mouth like oral thrush, loss of weight and diarrhoea.

People with HIV develop AIDS and will have episodes of opportunistic infections like tuberculosis, pneumonia, persistent diarrhoea, cancers and infections of the brain causing headaches, fits and mental confusion. Finally, the person cannot fight any more illnesses and dies.

HOW DOES HIV ENTER OUR BODY?

HIV can only enter our body through the ways shown in the box below. It cannot enter the body like the germs of other diseases, such as colds and diarrhoea.

HIV is found in large numbers in sexual fluids (such as vaginal secretions and semen) and blood. It is easy for HIV to enter through the thin lining (mucous membranes) of the vagina, penis, rectum and mouth where the mucous membrane is thin and the blood vessels are close to the surface.

BOX 1: WAYS IN WHICH HIV IS TRANSMITTED

- Through unprotected sexual intercourse (vaginal, anal or oral) with an infected person; that is, intercourse without a condom.
- Through contact with infected blood, for example by:
  - receiving a transmission of infected blood
  - the sharing of sharp skin-piercing instruments, such as injection needles that are not sterile
  - contact with open sores or wounds
- From an infected mother to her unborn or newly-born child

Ravi did not know that he was infected with HIV during sexual intercourse with Remani. The virus which was in the sexual fluids of Remani entered Ravi's body through the thin skin covering his penis. From the mucous membrane, the HIV entered the blood and his WBXs. When Ravi had sexual relationships with Radha, the HIV was passed from his sexual fluids into Radha's body through the thin lining of her vagina.

HIV infection is most often passed by unprotected sex. It can be passed from either a man or a woman when any type of sexual intercourse (vaginal, anal or oral) is performed without using a condom.

The virus was passed on to Kannan while he was in the womb.

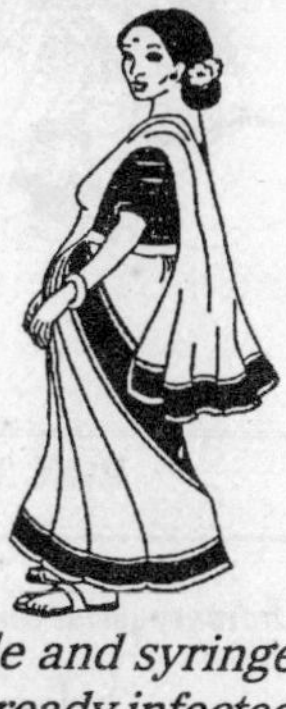

Infected mothers can pass the infection to their babies while in their womb or during childbirth or after childbirth through breast milk.

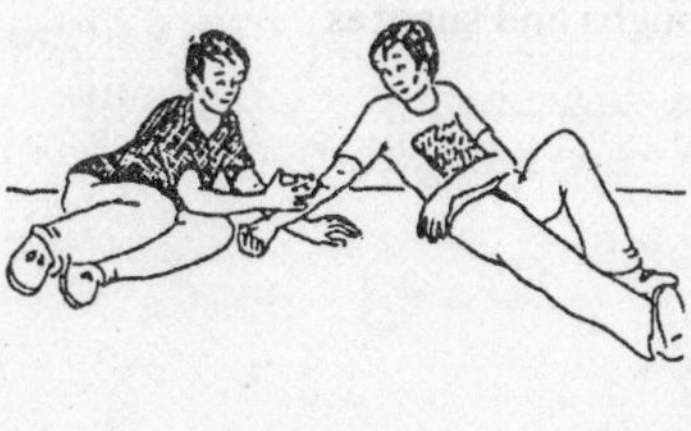

Mod shared a needle and syringe with Yut, who was already infected with HIV. The virus present in Yut's blood which was in the syringe and needle entered Mod's blood when he injected the drug using the same needle and syringe. Mod passed the infection to others in the hostel as they shared the same syringe and needle without cleaning them properly.

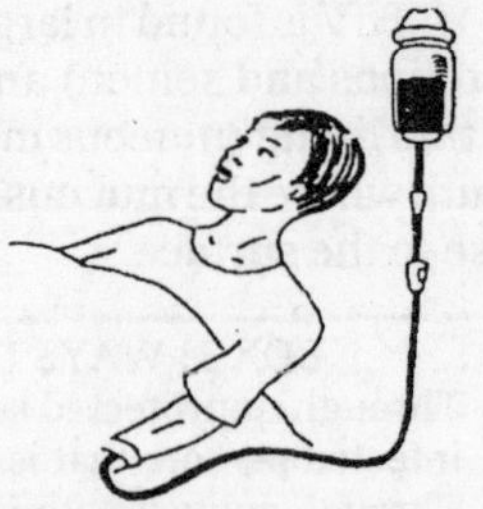

HIV is also passed through receiving infected blood or blood products or through the use of skin-piercing instruments which are contaminated.

Skin-piercing instruments like needles and syringes, instruments used for tattooing, piercing ears, etc., razor blades and instruments used by dentists and doctors, etc. if not sterilized properly can pass the infection to others. When an instrument or equipment which has been used on a person with HIV infection is used on another person without being sterilized or disinfected, then the virus which is in the blood left on the instrument enters the blood of the second person. Syringes and needles, especially, can carry the virus as there is always some blood or fluid stuck in the syringe which may not be easily visible.

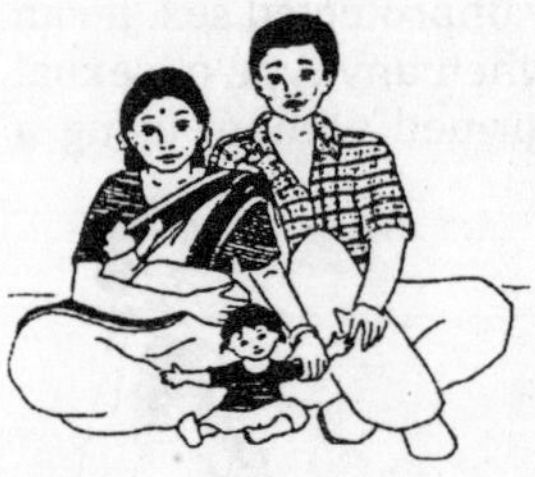

Meenakshi remains uninfected with HIV even though she has been living with three other members of the family who are infected with HIV. Meenakshi's contacts with her own family, the community, and her environment included many of the things listed in Box 2, but since there is no risk associated with these activities she did not get the virus. This is because HIV is not transmitted in these ways.

BOX 2: WAYS IN WHICH HIV IS NOT TRANSMITTED

Ordinary social contact:

- being physically close
  - in the same home
  - breathing the same air; coughs and sneezes
  - at work
  - on the bus
  - at the market
  - at school
  - playing together
- touching
  - shaking hands
  - hugging

— kissing on the cheeks, hands or forehead

Sharing:

- toilet seats
- towels
- washing water, bath water
- swimming pools
- eating and drinking utensils
- work tools

Being bitten by:

- mosquitoes
- bed bugs
- other insects
- any other animal

Donating blood

It is very important to understand that HIV is not spread through daily social contacts, at home, at work or in school. Otherwise, as people begin to see AIDS as a serious problem, they may panic and reject infected people. They may isolate them and their families. These reactions are deeply upsetting for people who are already facing the trauma of AIDS, and do not help stopping the transmission of HIV. If people are not encouraged to share the problems they have, then they cannot receive help from their families and enjoy the time they have together. For provision of care and to avoid the denial and stigmatization of AIDS, this information is crucial.

AIDS AND OTHER SEXUALLY TRANSMITTED DISEASES

Ravi had sores on his penis which became alright after he took treatment. This was an STD. Ravi got the disease that caused the sores during unprotected sexual intercourse with Remani. Remani got the sexually transmitted disease from one of her other sexual partners. The disease had damaged the surface of Remani's vagina which made it easy for HIV to enter her body and for her to pass it on to someone else during sexual intercourse. Ravi's chance of passing on HIV to Radha also increased after he developed the sores on his penis.

Sexually transmitted diseases (STDs) are also called venereal diseases. These diseases, as the name suggests, are spread through sexual intercourse:

- vaginal,
- anal, and
- oral

The germs which cause STDs can only enter the body through

the wet mucosal lining of the vagina, penis, rectum and mouth during sexual acts. They can also enter through the eyes if the eyes come in contact with the germs as in the case of newborns who get infected while passing through the birth canal during childbirth. The section on genital problems in Chapter Six gives more information on some of the STDs.

WHO IS AT RISK OF GETTING HIV?

Remani had multiple sex partners and she got the HIV infection from one of them. Ravi got infected with HIV when he had unprotected sex with Remani. He would not have got the HIV-infection if he had sexual intercourse only with Radha.

Mod is young and is curgous. He likes the company of his friends as he is away from home and is willing to do anything to please his friends. He got infected because Yut, with whom he shared the needle while injecting drugs, was infected with HIV.

Certain practices put people at risk and not what and who they are. For example, having unprotected sex with multiple partners puts one at greater risk. But a sex worker who practices protected/ safer sex is less at risk. Similarly, an injecting drug user who shares equipment is at greater risk, while the one who does not share or who sterilizes the equipment is less at risk. Examples: Adolescents, youth and street children are also at risk if they use drugs or have multiple sexual partners, which are more common among these groups.

Women with low social status and economic dependence may be sexually exploited and unable to negotiate safer sexual-practices. This makes them vulnerable to HIV infection. (See Chapter 4 for more information on Women, Children and HIV). People who regularly receive blood transfusions or other blood products are also at risk.

HOW CAN HIV AND AIDS BE AVOIDED?

Ravi got infected with HIV during sexual intercourse with Remani, then he passed the infection to Radha during sexual intercourse. How could Ravi avoid getting HIV infection and if he had known he was infected, how could he have avoided giving the infection to Radha?

A person who is not infected with HIV can take steps to avoid infection just as a person who is infected with HIV can take steps to prevent passing the HIV infection to someone else.

Prevention of transmission through sexual intercourse

Abstinence (not having sexual relations at all) is the surest way of preventing sexual transmission of HIV infection.

For many people, however, this may not be acceptable or realistic. The use of condoms and other safer sexual practices are the only ways of decreasing the risk of becoming infected with HIV or transmitting HIV infection to a sexual partner. Safer sexual practices are described in Box 3.

BOX 3 :WHAT IS SAFER SEX"?

"Safer sex" is any sexual practice that reduces the risk of passing (transmitting) HIV from one person to another.

The best protection is obtained by choosing sexual activities that do not allow semen, fluid from the vagina or blood to enter the mouth, anus or vagina of the partner, or to touch the skin of the partner where there is an open cut or sore.

Safer sex practices include:

- staying in a mutually faithful relationship where both partners are uninfected
- using a condom for all types of sexual intercourse (vaginal, anal or oral) so that the body secretions that contain HIV do not come in conduct with the skin or mucous membranes of the partner.
- avoiding penetrative sex, for example by replacing with: masturbation, massage, dry kissing, and hugging
- avoiding sex when either partner has open sores or a sexually transmitted disease (STD).

Couples should talk about safer sex and learn to please each other. This can make the intercourse more pleasurable for both and less likely to cause discomfort or minor damage to the genitals.

USE OF CONDOMS TO PREVENT HIV AND STD TRANSMISSION

Certainly, if Ravi had been faithful to his wife, this story might have been very different. Ravi could not have known if Remani was infected with HIV, and for that reason he should have used a condom. Use of condoms would have protected Ravi from getting the infection and passing it on to Radha. Ravi could have avoided getting the STD and HIV if he had used condoms while having sexual intercourse with Remani. Prevention of STDs could have reduced the risk of Remani getting infected with HIV.

Condoms are the most effective means of protection against the organisms that cause sexually transmitted diseases, including HIV.

Condoms are effective only if they are used properly during every sexual intercourse. Instructions on how to use condoms are given in Box 4.

BOX 4 HOW TO USE A CONDOM?

- Be sure you have a condom before you need it.
- Each time you have sex put a new and unused condom on the penis before it enters the vagina, rectum or mouth.
- Put the condom on only when the penis is erect.
- When putting on the condom, hold it so that the rolled rim is on the outside. If you are not circumcised, first pull the foreskin of the penis back.
- Do not pull the condom tightly against the tip of the penis but pinch the end of the condom when unrolling it this leaves a small empty space, to hold the semen.
- Unroll the condom all the way to the base of the penis.
- If the condom tears during sex, withdraw the penis immediately and put on a new condom.
- After ejaculation, hold on to the bottom of the condom as you pull the penis out, so that the condom does not slip off, then take off the condom carefully without spilling semen.
- Wrap the condom in paper (such as newspaper) until you can dispose of it in a toilet, a pit latrine, or a closed garbage bag, or by burying or burning it.

The following tips will help prevent condoms breaking or leaking.

- If lubricant is needed, use a water-based one (like KY Jelly, or glycerine). Do not use a lubricant made with oil, like Vaseline.
- Store condoms in a cool, dark, dry place. Heat, light and humidity can damage condoms.
- If you have a choice, choose pre-lubricated condoms that are packaged so that light does not reach them.
- Open the wrapper carefully so that the condom does not tear.
- Do not use condoms that are sticky, brittle, discoloured or damaged in any way.

Remember! Correct and consistent use of condoms will protect you from HIV.

Drawings or teaching models can be very helpful in teaching people how to use condoms correctly. The types of instructions, drawings and models available for this purpose vary from country to country. You can use the written instructions provided in the above box to accompany any pictures or models you are using. A sample illustration is given here below:

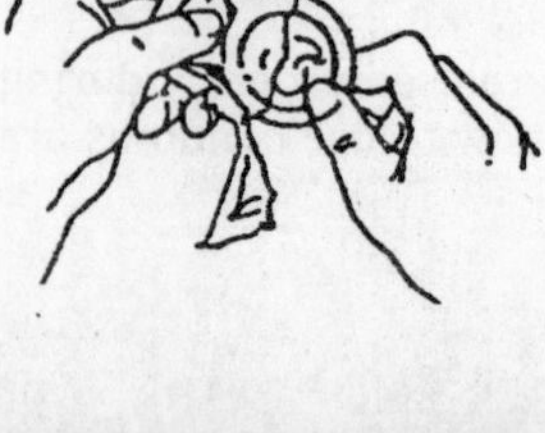

Carefully open the package so the condom does not tear. Do not unroll condom before putting it on.

If not circumcised, pull foreskin back. Squeeze tip of condom and put it on end of hard penis.

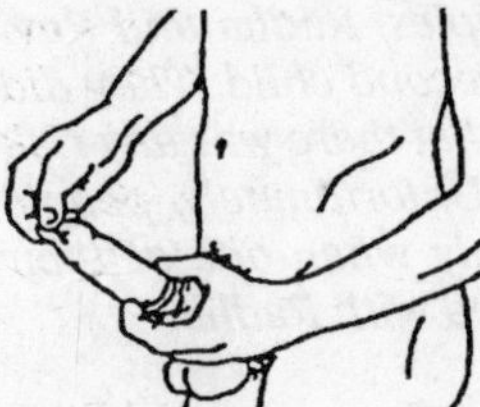

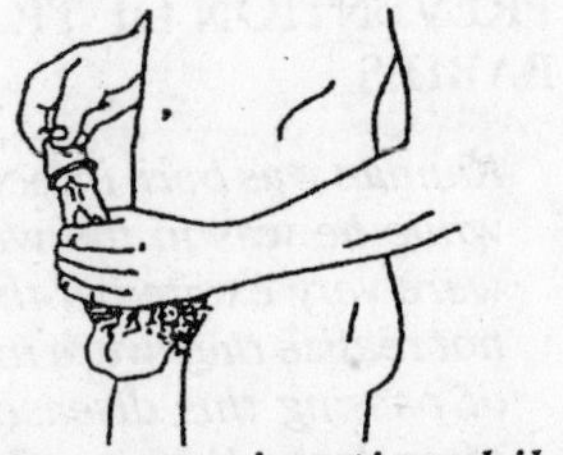

Continue squeezing tip while unrolling condom until it covers all of penis.

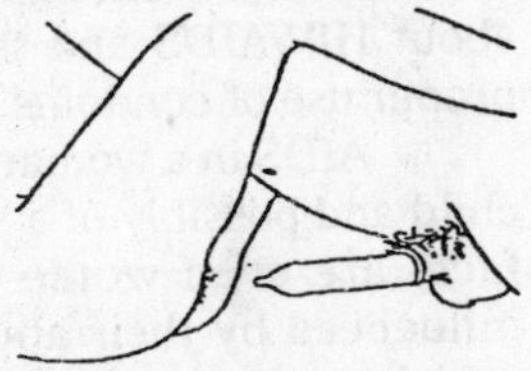

Always put on a condom before entering partner.

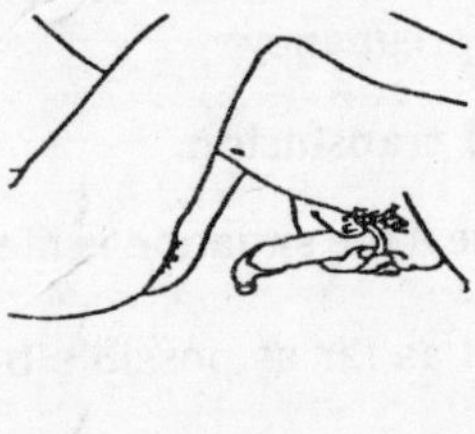

After ejaculation hold rim of condom and pull penis out before penis gets soft.

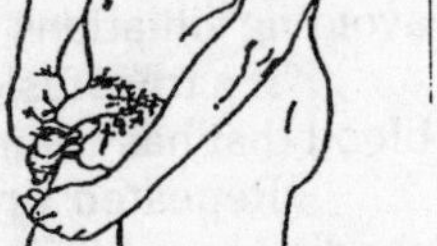

Slide condom off without spilling liquid (semen) inside.

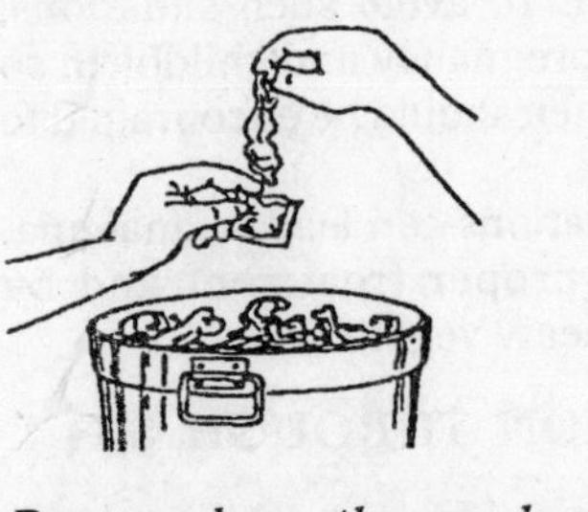

Tie and wrap the condom (in paper, if available) then throw in dust bin. Wash

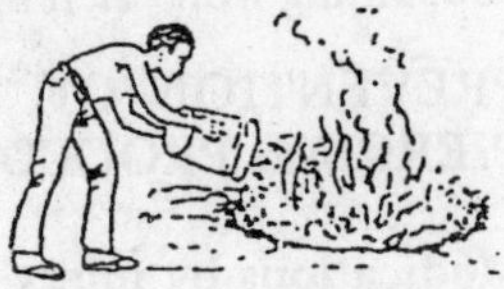

Burn or bury the condom with other trash. Wash hands.

PREVENTION OF TRANSMISSION FROM MOTHERS TO BABIES

Kannan was born infected with HIV. He probably got the infection while he was in the womb. Like most couples, Radha and Ravi were very excited at the idea of having a second child. They did not realize they were infected with HIV or that there was any risk of passing this disease on to their child. Unfortunately, people often learn they are infected with HIV only when one of their children becomes ill with AIDS as happened with Radha.

Prevention of sexual transmission of HIV to women is the best way to prevent this mode of transmission. Women should know about HIV/AIDS and that HIV transmission can be prevented by proper use of condoms.

AIDS in a woman brings with it the risk of having an infected child and possibly of a worsening of her own illness. These painful facts are even worse in places where the status of women is influenced by their ability to bear children and where it may be socially unacceptable or very difficult to take the necessary steps to avoid pregnancy - abstain from sexual intercourse or use contraception - or to consider terminating a pregnancy.

Prevention of transmission through blood transfusion.

Blood transfusions should only be done if the situation is life-threatening.

Blood transfusions should be avoided as far as possible by avoiding situations requiring them.

If a transfusion cannot be avoided, then one should insist on blood that has been tested for the presence of HIV antibodies.

Repeated pregnancies cause anaemia, which can lead to conditions requiring blood transfusion. To avoid such situations, women should get proper care during pregnancy and childbirth so that complications can be avoided. Women should be encouraged to eat foods rich in iron during pregnancy.

Malaria and certain worm infestations can lead to anaemia. Anaemia can be avoided by taking proper treatment and by consuming iron - rich foods like green leafy vegetables.

PREVENTION OF TRANSMISSION THROUGH SKIN-PIERCING PROCEDURES

Medications by injection

- All injections should be avoided as far as possible. Oral medication should be used if possible.
- If injections cannot be avoided, make sure that the needles

and syringes are either new disposable ones or are boiled or sterilized.

Addictive drugs by injection

- It is best to avoid all addictive drugs.
- If not possible, it is better to use them orally.
- If injecting drugs cannot be avoided, then injecting equipment should not be shared.

If not possible to avoid sharing injecting equipment, then either boil the equipment for 20 minutes or use bleach in the following manner:

- A level teaspoon of household bleach should be mixed with a litre of clean water in a bowl
- flush the syringe and needle first with water and only then flush the syringe and needle twice with the bleach solution
- flush the syringe and needle twice with water.
- Boil or disinfect all insheuments used for ear piercing, tattooing, circumcision, cutting the skin, sharing, etc.
- Do not share shaving razors or knives

HIV TESTING

Unfortunately, neither Ravi nor Radha understood the disease or the importance of HIV testing. A blood test for HIV in the first three months after HIV has entered the body can be negative ("the window period"). This is because the test for HIV infection looks for antibodies produced against HIV and not for the virus itself. Only after these antibodies are made will an HIV test be positive, even though the virus is present throughout this initial period (see Box 5).

The mild illness that Radha experienced at that time could have been caused by her initial infection with HIV. Most people experience a mild flu-like illness a few weeks after they become infected.

Shortly after her initial infection with HIV, Radha's body responded to the virus by making antibodies against it.

Now her test would be positive because she has antibodies to the virus in her blood.

WHO SHOULD GET AN HIV TEST AND WHEN?

HIV testing is recommended only if:

- someone is concerned that they may be infected because:
  - of unprotected sex
  - of transfusion with untested blood
  - of sharing needles or other injection equipment
- one of the sexual partners is infected.

BOX 5: HIV TESTING

What is an HIV test?

Shortly after infection with HIV, the body starts to respond by making antibodies against the virus. This usually takes about 6-12 weeks. An HIV test is a blood test that can find out if these specific antibodies are present in the blood it does not detect the virus itself.

What do the results mean?

- A positive result in a person over 15 months old means that:

- the person has antibodies against HIV, and is thus HIV-infected and can transmit the virus to others (see Box 1).

- A positive result in a child under 5 months old can mean either that:
    - the child is infected with HIV, or
    - the child is not infected with HIV, but has received antibodies from the mother, in the same way as many other antibodies are transferred during pregnancy.
- A negative test result can mean either that:
    - the person is not infected with HIV, or
    - the person is infected with HIV, but has not yet made antibodies against the virus. (This is called the "window period".)
- The HIV test
    - does not provide any information about a person's present state of health
    - does not determine if a person has HIV-related disease
    - cannot tell when or how a person became infected with HIV
    - does not tell if a person with HIV infection has transmitted the virus to anyone else.

Because the results of the HIV test can have dramatic effects on families relationships, employment and the individual's own well-being, it is important that people be tested only with their consent, that they be counselled before and after testing, and that the results be kept confidential, that is, shared only with the individual, or others designated by the individual

3

Living Positively with AIDS

Living positively with AIDS means taking care of one's health, leading an active life in society and living in a responsible manner so that the infection is not passed on to others. Positive living requires the families and communities to support HIV-positive people for a life with dignity and love.

This chapter tells the second part of Story 1 about AIDS, which is again followed by teaching notes providing more information. The story continues from where it left off in Chapter 2, and is presented again in a way that you can use directly when teaching.

THE NEXT PART OF THE STORY–RADHA AND MEENAKSHI

- **Let us join Radha and her family again, where we left off before.**

EARLY 1993

Radha's husband has just died and she makes a few plans for the future. Radha has picked up courage during Ravi's illness and, with the support of her family, has grown in strength. She resolves to remain healthy and emotionally strong for Meenakshi.

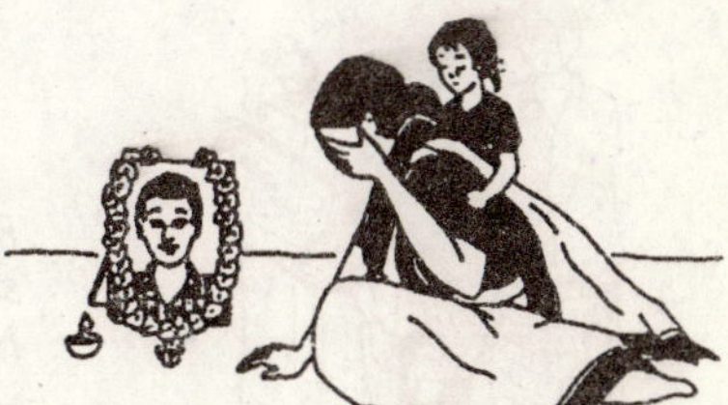

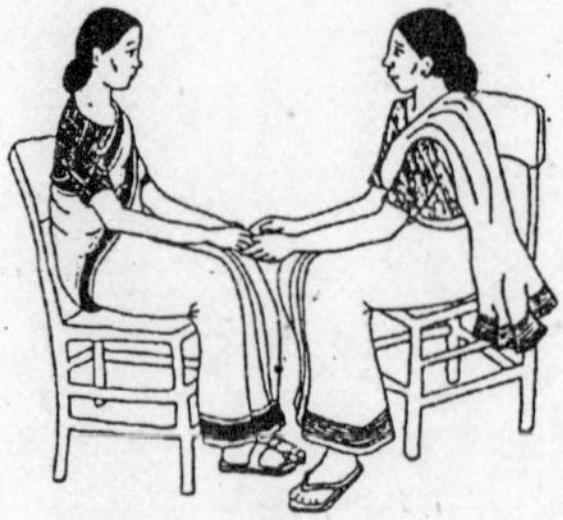

Radha remembers the words of Kannan's doctor and wonders whether Ravi also died of AIDS. She decides to get herself tested to see whether she has the same illness. After the traditional period of mourning is over, Radha goes to a clinic for a HIV blood test. A 'counsellor' talks with her for a long time about her life and what the test means. A small sample of her blood is taken and she is asked to come to the clinic after a few days.

Radha returns to the clinic and meets the counsellor who tells her that the test is positive which means that she is infected with the virus. Radha is shocked. She bursts out crying. The counsellor is very kind and talks to Radha for a long time. She tells Radha that she must come to terms with and accept that she has HIV, and live as long as she can for Meenakshi's sake. She explains what HIV and AIDS are, and how they are transmitted and prevented. The counsellor tells her that there are many things she can do, and that there are many people who will help her. She also tells Radha that there are many other people who are infected with HIV and how some of them are helping her in the clinic and also visiting homes of people who are sick and providing help.

Radha decides that she must start earning to support herself and Meenakshi. With the help of Ravi's colleagues in the factory, Radha gets some refund for the medical expenses incurred for Ravi's treatment as well as the money due to him from the employee's fund. Radha decides to open a small shop with some of the money. She puts some money in the bank for Meenakshi.

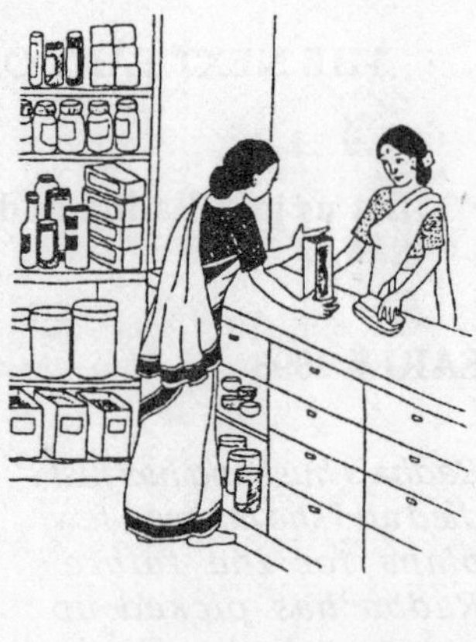

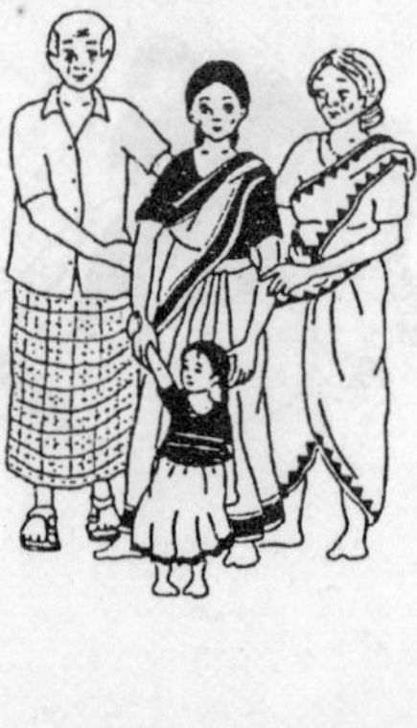

Radha's parents have been a source of strength for her. They have come to stay with Radha for sometime.

MID-1993

At times Radha does not feel well and she goes to the clinic for treatment. Her father helps out in the shop when she is not well. Radha has been earning enough from the shop to support herself and Meenakshi. During one of Radha's visits to the clinic, she sees a young woman crying. Radha wants to console her, but does not feel confident. The young girl's face haunts Radha for many days. She realizes that there may be many people like her who need help. She decides to help such people. She discusses this with her parents who agree to take care of the shop and Meenakshi while she is away. She goes to the clinic and meets the counsellor and tells her that she would like to help out in the clinic in the afternoons.

The counsellor promises to give her some training. She gets trained to provide support to those who are HIV-positive, and to help those who are sick, especially with AIDS.

LATE 1993

Radha visits people in their homes. She sometimes takes Meenakshi with her and she helps with simple chores.

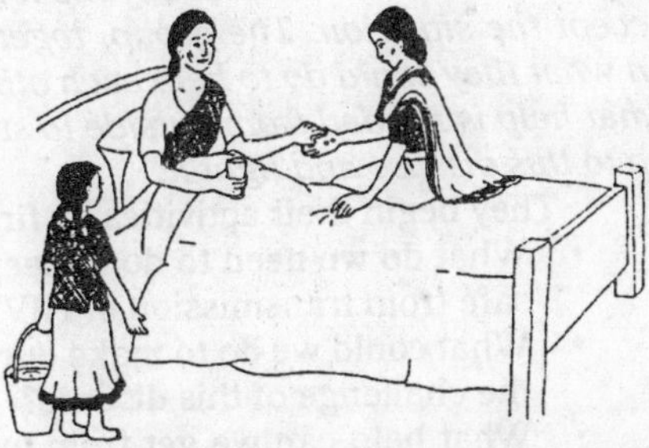

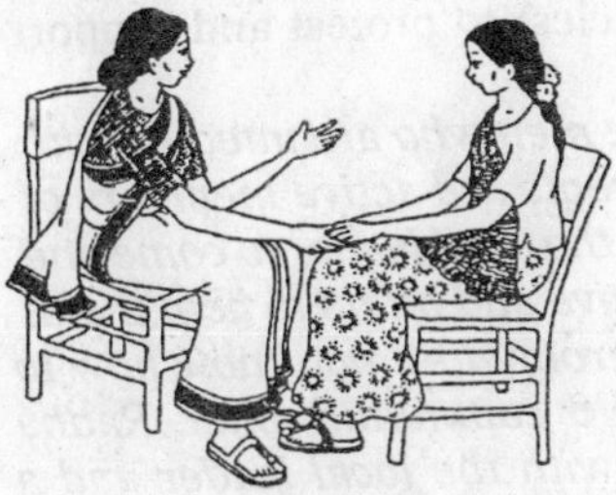

Radha also counsels people who are infected with HIV. She talks in the community about preventing the spread of HIV infection. She gives both her knowledge and her hope. She says she can live positively with AIDS and that when she dies the virus in her will die too.

Radha discovers that the families of these people are facing many difficulties - as the story shows, these can be emotional, social and economic difficulties. In families where the husbands have died due to AIDS or are ill due to AIDS, women have to work hard outside their homes to earn something to feed and look after the family. The children in these families are affected in many ways. Often, there is not enough food for all— Children stop going to school because their families can't afford the expenses or they stay back to take care of their younger sisters or brothers.

Radha is very concerned about what is happening in her community. She had heard during her training that in some communities there is help for people with AIDS practical and spiritual help, help with ways to make money, keep jobs, find food and medicines, make wills and ensure that last wishes are respected.

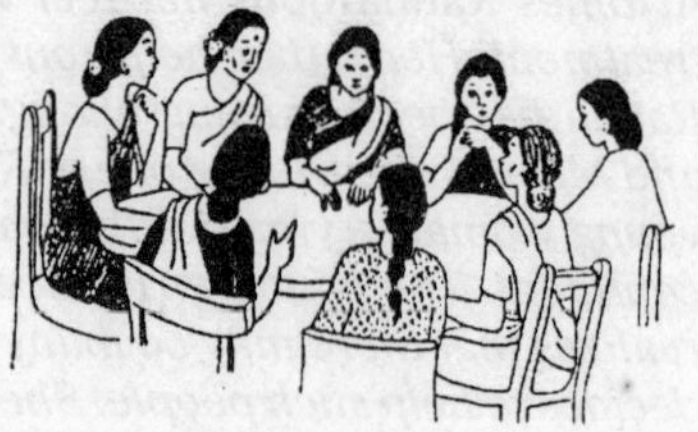

She wants to organize similar activities in her community, so she shares her ideas with the women. Some of these women are infected with HIV and some are from families of people infected with HIV.

The group shares their experiences, concerns and sorrows. They decide not to find fault with anyone for bringing the infection. They accept the situation. The group, together, starts making decisions on what they could do to help each other and their community, and what help is needed from outside to strengthen their ability to face up to this disease and fight it.

They begin their activities by first asking themselves:

- What do we need to do to keep ourselves and our families safe from transmission of HIV?
- What could we do to make our community stronger to face the challenge of this disease?
- What help can we get from outside our community (from the government or other agencies) to protect and support our people?

The group slowly expands to include men who are infected with HIV and others as well. Radha's parents are active members of the group. One day, the group invites the local leader to come and join them. The leader is very supportive and offers to help them.

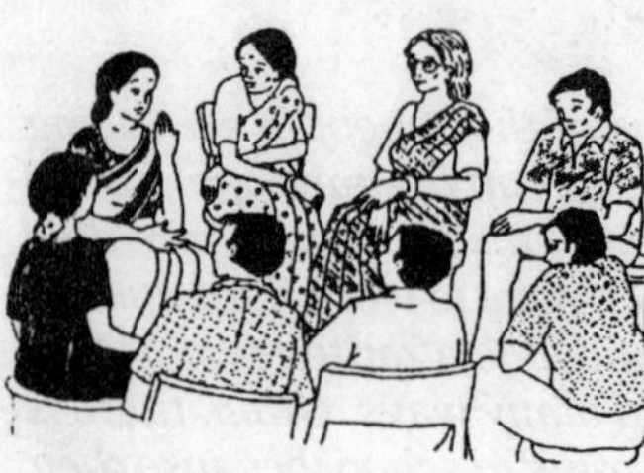

The group does not know how to make a community plan. Radha goes with the local leader and a few others to the people who had given her training and they offer to come and help the group Radha had organized. Together with these people, the group makes a community plan. Together they begin to collect money, small amounts left over from what they have, and to set it aside for the children.

They form a support group, talk openly and share information about AIDS and how to prevent its spread in their community. They arrange for some materials for the sick from local voluntary organizations. The face of the community changes. It becomes a friendlier place in which to live and die.

LATE 1994

Getting timely health care for people with AIDS has been a problem. Radha and some of the members of the organization meet the local health centre staff and discuss their problems. The staff tell them that it may be difficult to provide care in all the homes in the area They tell them that they will be happy to provide training to family members who can then provide care at home and refer problems to the health centre.

TEACHING NOTES ON LIVING POSITIVELY WITH AIDS

Responses to AIDS

Each of these feelings or reactions is part of a normal response to a situation of great stress. A person might move from one response to the next in a progression leading finally to acceptance of their situation, or more commonly their feelings will keep changing. Some days they might feel rejected and lonely and others hopeful and energetic, one day depressed, another day angry. Let us look at each of these reactions separately and think about how these make someone feel, and how a person feeling like this might be helped.

Take the audience back to the story and look in detail how Radha coped with the deaths of Kannan and Ravi. As in Chapter 2, the information is presented below in a way you can use directly when teaching.

Radha was shocked when Kannan's doctor told her about AIDS and that he suspected that Kannan had AIDS. Her reaction in such a situation was normal.

Mod was shocked to hear that his HIV test was positive.

When somebody experiences a shock or a loss they have feelings or emotions called "loss reactions". These are feelings which come when new and serious problems like HIV and AIDS are confronted. It is normal to have strong feelings about them. Most people are frightened of HIV and AIDS.

Radha refused to believe that Kannan had AIDS. Radha was not convinced that Kannan got the HIV infection while he was in her womb, thereby refusing to believe that she could be infected. Even though she got herself tested, she never went back to find out the results of the test. She never discussed with Ravi what the doctor had told her - maybe because she didn't believe what the doctor had said or she was afraid of Ravi's reactions. The doctor had told her how HIV infection is transmitted and she didn't want to believe that Ravi could have had sexual intercourse with someone else.

People who find out that they have HIV infection or AIDS, or learn that someone important to them has HIV or AIDS, may experience many different feelings such as anger, fear and sadness. Sometimes, people may deny having the disease at all. Feelings of denial can cause family communications to break down.

Ravi's illness and eventually his death made Radha realize the facts that both Kannan and Ravi died of AIDS and that she may be infected. She decided to go for a second test to find out whether she was infected. When she found out that her test was positive, she decided that she must do everything possible to provide proper care to Meenakshi. She also started helping others in the community who are infected with HIV or have AIDS. She also organized the community to provide support and care to those infected with HIV or those with AIDS.

Mod accepted the fact that he was infected with HIV and decided to live positively and help others who are infected with HIV.

Denial, unfortunately, is a very common reaction which delays positive action. Only after getting over this reaction and accepting the situation can any positive action start.

- **What may have been the reason for Radha's denial?**

Radha didn't want to go back to find out the results of her first test. She was probably afraid that if her test was positive, Ravi may leave her. She didn't know how her friends and neighbours would react. She was concerned about Meenakshi s future - whether she would be refused admission in the school.

- **Even though Radha had accepted the fact that Kannan and Ravi died of AIDS and that, most probably, she was infected, she was shocked when she heard that her test was positive.**

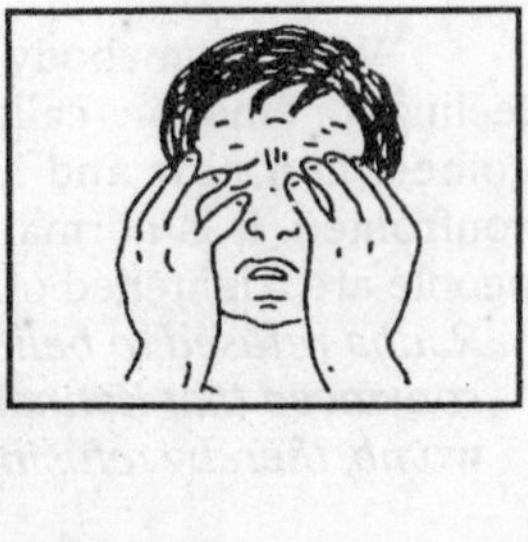

How would you have reacted if you were told that you have HIV infection?

SHOCK

No matter how much someone is prepared, it is a shock to learn that one has HIV infection or AIDS. A person might feel confused and not know what to do. It is good for people to be with someone they trust at this time.

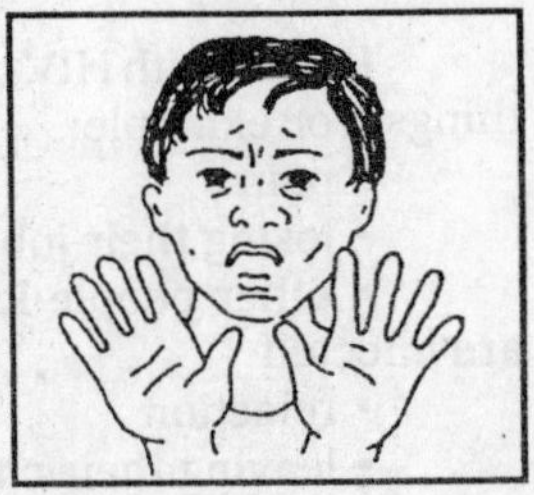

DENIAL

At first they might not be able to believe that they really have HIV or AIDS. They might think, "The doctor must be wrong" or "It can't be true I feel so strong". Not wanting to believe is a strong force that people may use subconsciously to protect themselves from the threat posed by AIDS. Denial may come from the fear of being rejected by loved ones. If you are trying to help such people, don't be angry or impatient with them if it seems that they are not facing facts. Try to remember that as a provider of care you can help them to understand how they became infected, what having HIV or AIDS means and that this is the best way to help overcome denial.

ANGER

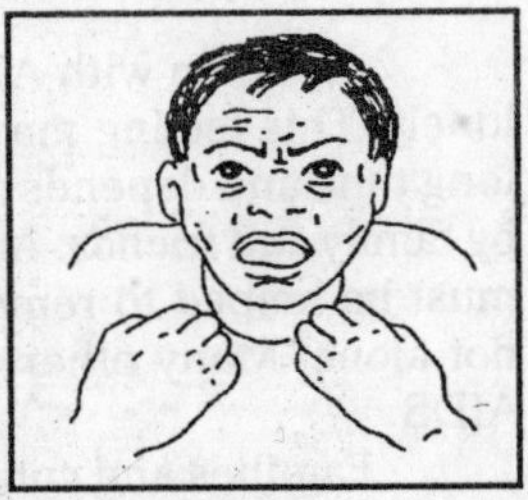

People might become very angry when they learn that they have HIV or AIDS. This is a common feeling and can come when they blame themselves or the person they think gave them HIV Some may even blame God.

Anger is normal but it may not be helpful since it can focus on blaming others (being angry with them) or themselves (feeling guilty), rather than taking positive actions. Talking to someone can help a person overcome feelings of anger and help them accept their situation.

If you are trying to help someone with HIV or AIDS, anger is a difficult reaction to cope with, especially when it is directed at you. It is important for you to try to understand and not take the anger personally. It is difficult, of course, to receive anger without responding.

BARGAINING

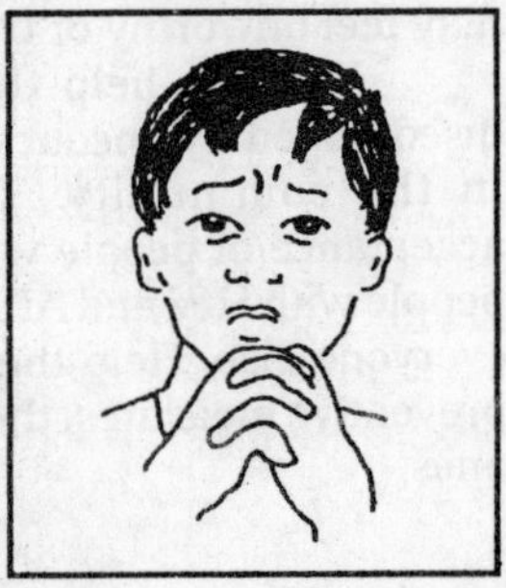

A person with AIDS might try to bargain, thinking, "God will cure me if I stop having sex" or "The ancestors will make me better if I slaughter a goat" or "I will be good and it (AIDS) will go away". People with HIV or AIDS need to be helped to accept reality.

FEAR

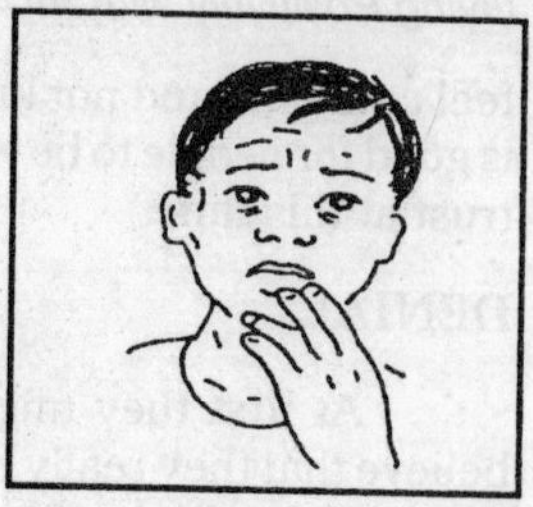

People with HIV or AIDS fear many things. For example:

- pain
- losing their job
- other people knowing that they are infected
- relection .
- leaving their children
- the future of their family
- death.

The fears become less when they talk to someone who understands. Those with AIDS might also find that they are worried about things that they do not need to fear. For example, they may find that when other people learn they have HIV, they show great love and kindness rather than the feared rejection.

LONELINESS

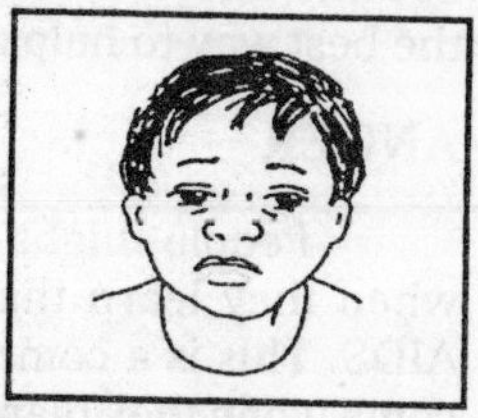

A person with AIDS might often feel lonely. This feeling may come and go for a long time and depends on the support given by family and friends. Anyone who has AIDS must be helped to remember that they are not alone. Many other people have HIV or AIDS.

Families and communities must understand that people with HIV and AIDS need companionship, especially of people not infected with HIV. Infected people can often find others with HIV and AIDS and provide companionship and support for one another.

SELF-CONSCIOUSNESS

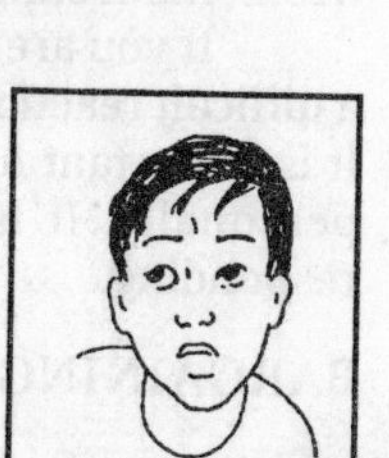

People with HIV or AIDS might think everyone is looking at them or talking about them even though this is not the case. This may make them want to hide. Sometimes a person with AIDS may feel unworthy of friendship.

You can help them not to hide or feel discouraged by encouraging them to stay active in the community. This can increase the acceptance of people with HIV or AIDS by showing the world that people with HIV and AIDS are valuable members of society, just like everyone else. Help them to understand that as long as they take preventive measures, they will not spread the infection to their loved ones.

Help them to think well of themselves and to be proud. They are as important as everyone else.

DEPRESSION

If someone finds out that they have HIV or AIDS, they may feel there is no good reason for living. They may feel useless, and want to stay at home, not eat, and not talk to anyone.

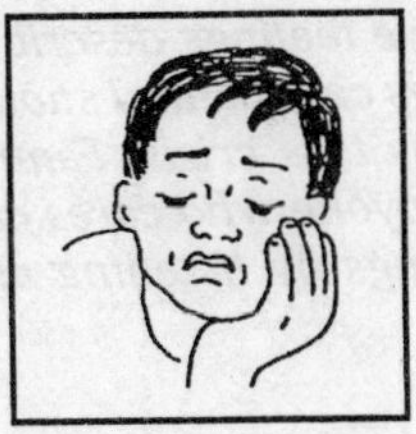

Depression can make someone weak both in mind and body. It is important to try and help them overcome this depression and not give up. Encourage them to continue with their normal routine as well as to put on nice clothes, visit friends, keep busy with things that matter, do something that helps others, and to think about their children and friends who still need them.

ACCEPTANCE

After some time, people with HIV or AIDS will usually begin to accept their situation. This helps them to feel better. Such persons will feel more peaceful, and will begin to think about the best ways to live.

They might think:

- "What can I do to make the best of the rest of my life?"
- "What foods should I eat to help me stay healthy?"
- What plans should I make so that my children are provided for in the future?"
- "Let me be grateful for every single day. Let me appreciate my family and friends and show them how much I care for them."

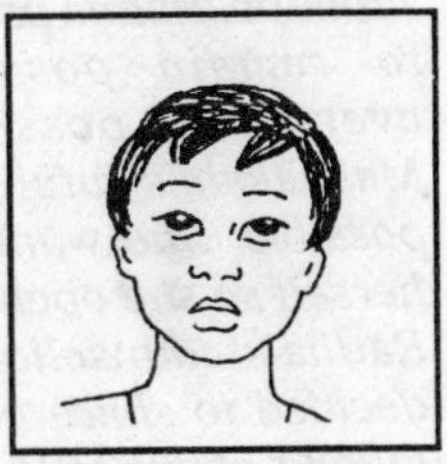

HOPE

You can help someone with HIV or AIDS have hope about many things.

For example:

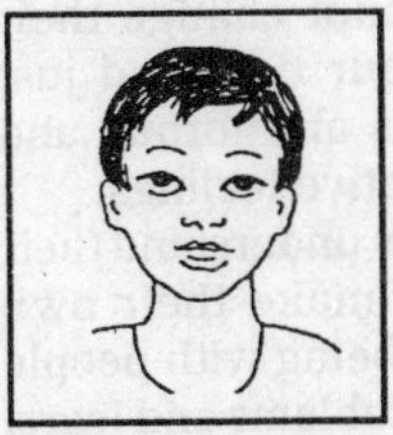

- hope that they will live a long time
- hope that their baby will be healthy
- hope that each sickness will be treated as it comes
- hope that they are loved and accepted for who they are
- hope that scientists will find a cure
- hope based on belief in a life after death.

It is important to have hope. Hope lifts spirits and gives strength to face each situation. Hope can help each person to fight HIV and AIDS to live positively and to live longer.

Remember, even if a person has hope today, it is possible to feel angry or depressed tomorrow. This is normal. Even people without HIV or AIDS go up and down emotionally every day. The important thing is to try to instill the feelings of hope again and again.

People who have AIDS, or people who are in contact with someone with AIDS, are often afraid that the negative feelings described above will become too strong. These feelings cannot, and should not, be avoided. They are normal reactions to a crisis. Family, friends, neighbours, health care workers anyone who cares can help another person cope with these feelings by listening and talking to the person about their feelings.

WHAT IS COUNSELLING?

After Ravi's death, when Radha went back to get her HIV test done, the counsellor in the clinic talked with her. Radha's counsellor helped her to accept the fact that she is infected with HIV and helped her to cope with the situation. Radha promised herself to remain positive and do everything possible to make Meenakshi's future as secure as possible. She wanted to support herself so she opened a shop.

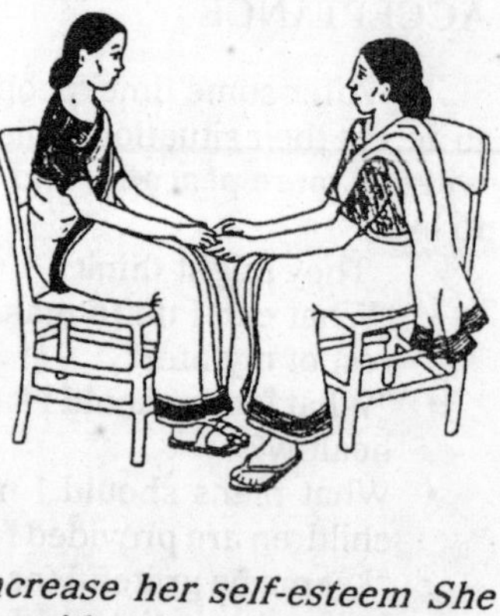

Radha's counsellor helped her to increase her self-esteem She decided to share her positive feelings with others, so she started talking about HIV prevention and visiting those who are infected with HIV in the community.

Counselling helped Mod to take decisions himself about quitting use of injecting drugs. Mod was able to live positively and provide care and support to other injecting drug users infected with HIV.

In the previous section, you saw the reactions people might have on learning that they are infected with HIV or have AIDS. No matter how much you care for people you cannot change their feelings. Only they can do that. By offering your time and just listening, you are telling them that their feelings are normal and accepted, and you help them overcome their negative feelings.

Counsellors are people trained to help others understand their problems, identify and develop solutions, and make their own decisions about what to do. Counselling involves being with people with problems, listening to them talk about their problems and fears.

helping them to increase their own self-esteem, and when necessary giving *correct* and *useful* information based on what they need to know at this point in time.

Many of the skills needed for counselling are similar to those needed for teaching (see Chapter 1), because they are skills of effective *communication.*

Counselling is a skill that requires effective training to develop. There may be times, if you are working with people with HIV or AIDS and their families, when you believe more skilled counselling is needed to deal with serious psychological issues. At these times you may want to refer the sick person for help elsewhere, from people who are experienced in providing such support, perhaps in government or voluntary services or in religious or spiritual organizations.

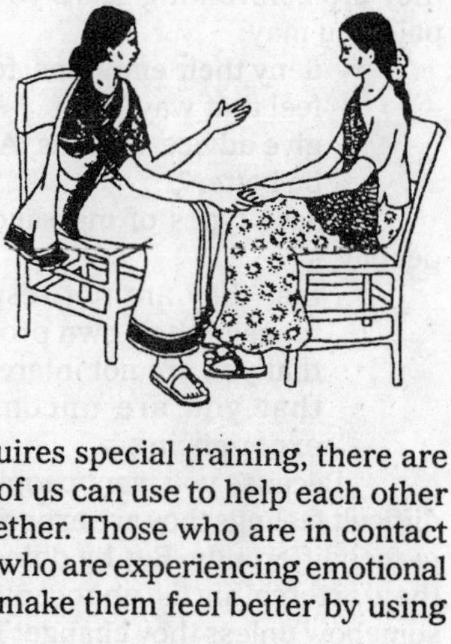

Radha was taught simple counseling techniques during her training. This helped her to help people infected with HIV or with AIDS. Her efforts helped many to take positive actions.

Even though counselling requires special training, there are skills used by counsellors which all of us can use to help each other during the times we are talking together. Those who are in contact with people with AIDS, or with those who are experiencing emotional pain, can do a lot to help them and make them feel better by using simple counselling techniques.

- **Think of a time when you felt badly about something and how, after talking with someone else a friend, a family member, a health care worker, a religious leader you felt better. What did that other person do that "helped" you? Can you remember?**

Often the answer is:

"Nothing, he just listened and sat with me while I told him everything."

Or maybe:

"She was just kind and didn't judge anything I said. She helped me to understand what was really bothering me and what I could do."

These answers tell us what some of these effective communication skills are:

- listening actively
- trying to understand what the person is feeling
- asking good questions
- respecting people and their feelings, and not telling them to change
- being non-judgemental
- providing correct information

All these things tell a person, "You are not alone. I am with you". This is important to someone who is afraid of being rejected and who might feel like a failure.

The most common mistake you can make when trying to "help" people who are experiencing emotional pain is to try to change their feelings. You don't want them to be hurt and perhaps the issues they are confronting scare you too. To distance yourself from this pain you may:

- deny their emotions, for example by saying, "You shouldn't feel that way".
- give advice, such as "All you need to do is ... and things will be better".

These types of messages are a "mistake" because they tell people:

- that they are not respected or capable that they cannot manage their own problems
- that you are not interested in them or their problems
- that you are uncomfortable with the pain they are experiencing.

Because you want people to feel better or to be "cured" of the difficult feelings they are experiencing, you may try to-convince them to feel differently. But by doing this you are telling them that what they are feeling is unacceptable and that they are failing you somehow unless they change. This only adds to their feelings of self-rejection and isolation.

Listening is one of the most important parts of good communication. This means you have to be silent sometimes. Let the conversation move at the other person's speed rather than at yours.

Asking good questions comes from good listening and is part of helping someone see another point of view. The questions you ask should always come from your listening. When you listen you are not just hearing words, you are hearing the feelings behind the words and the person's own view of their situation. The questions you ask can help both of you gain a better understanding of the situation.

Another important way you can help is by being able to give consistent and accurate information. The ability to say you do not know an answer but will try to find one is *always* better than making an answer up (see Chapter 1). Telling the truth establishes the trust and the respect needed to build a helpful relationship.

The trust you earn means you must guard the privacy of the information shared. Never gossip or break this trust. Breaking trust tells a person:

- they are not worthy of respect
- it was a mistake to seek help or share their feelings

Further repercussions can include:

- the person may become withdrawn and avoid meeting others they think know their HIV status
- rumours may spread since pcople may not be familiar with HIV infection.

Because of this, they may not seek the help they need in the future.

There are often no easy answers to some of the difficult questions that are asked by those with HIV infection or AIDS. You cannot always have the "right" answer. Using truth and your ability to care are the only things you can be certain are right~. Your own discomfort and fears will be part of your attempts to help. Sometimes you will need to pay attention to these feelings and get help for yourself Perhaps this comment from a woman who described the counselling she reachieved says it all equally well:

"He looked me in the eye and said, "I don't know what I would do in your situation) except I would be scared". I felt, suddenly, so much better. I was scared but I wasn't alone somehow."

When you are caring for someone you must watch your own reactions to the person you are trying to help. If you find yourself becoming an patient or angry these are signs that you are having trouble dealing with your own emotions and are less likely to be helpful to the person. You may be thinking, "He just doesn't seem to be able to face facts" or "She won't do anything to help herself. Your needs as a care provider cannot be ignored but they should not be a burden to the person who is experiencing the grief of his or her own condition. You may need some special time to address your own concerns in private with counsellors, religious leaders or other providers of care. You may need help in understanding the sick person's needs and fears. You may just need a rest.

As AIDS wotsens and a person becomes more and more ill, very often worries about physical health are outweighed by practical and emotional worries about money, housing, disability, change in lifestyle, family and other relationships, and the approach of death. You can help by offering practical help in planning for the future and by giving spiritual support, for example by helping someone strengthen or re-establish their religious affiliation (see Chapter 5).

IMPORTANCE OF THE FAMILY

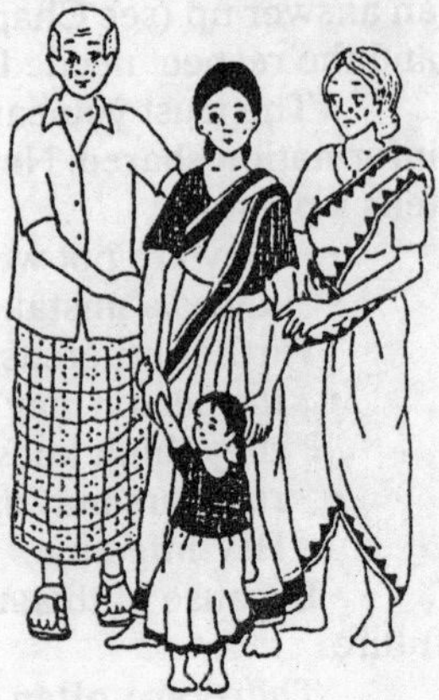

Radha had a lot of help from her parents. They gave her emotional support. They assisted her in running the shop as well as in taking care of Meenakshi. They encouraged her to undergo the training so that she could help others. They also played a major role in organizing community support.

Families are very important for people with HIV infection or AIDS and they can help them to live positively.

The family home can be a shelter:

- where a person is assured that he or she is loved and accepted
- where one doesn't have to hide one's feelings
- where one won't feel isolated.

If a person has HIV infection or AIDS, it is good for the family to know about it. This will enable the family:

- to give emotional support, love and care
- to help with daily chores in times of sickness
- to help make plans for the future
- to share some of the financial burden
- to prevent further HIV transmission.

The person with HIV/AIDS also has an opportunity to teach the family members about HIV infection and how to protect themselves from it.

COMMUNITY SUPPORT

Radha and Meenakshi going into the homes of other people with AIDS gave a very important message in the community.

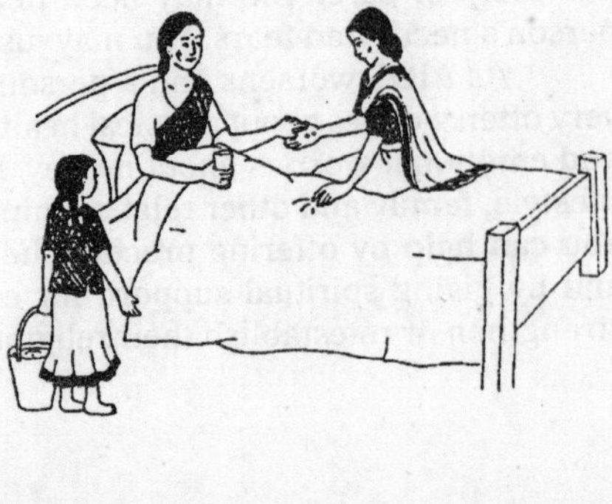

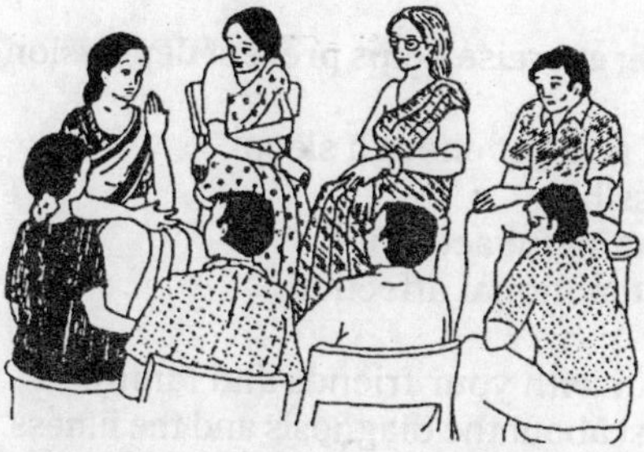

Radha played a major role in helping the community to provide care for those who are infected with HIV or have AIDS. The support group tried to identify local organizations and institutions that could help them. They coordinated their health care activities with the existing health institutions and also arranged for training in home care. These efforts changed the face of Radha's community and it became a community which is more caring and supportive.

Communities have a major role to play in care and support of people with HIV infection or AIDS. Communities should be encouraged to organize care and support to people infected with HIV or AIDS and to their families. They should be encouraged to make full use of the existing prograrnmes of the government and nongovernmental organizations in health and social sectors. For example, these organizations can train community workers, who may be family members or volunteers.

Often the help needed in caring for someone with AIDS and for those who love them is very simple. Offering to help with chores, bringing favourite foods, watching over children and playing with them, telling stories, singing songs, sharing prayers these are simple acts with strong; messages of hope and belonging.

WHAT EVERYONE WITH HIV OR AIDS SHOULD KNOW

- **Radha was told many things about HIV and AIDS by the counsellor who gave her the results of her HIV test.**

First, it is currently believed that all people with HIV infection will go on to develop AIDS. Modern medicine and traditional healers do not yet have a cure for AIDS. People who develop AIDS on average live for 1-2 years after symptoms appear, depending on a number of factors including nutritional status, access to health care and emotional support. But, many of the infections that come with AIDS can be treated and many symptoms can be dealt with by using simple medicines and proper care. Most importantly Radha was taught about how to live positively with AIDS. She learned that if you have HIV or AIDS you should try to keep strong. This means you should:

- eat as well as possible, with a mixture of staple foods, peas and beans, leafy dark green and orange vegetables, fruits, and oils and fats.

- stay as active as possible; exercise helps prevent depression and anxiety.
- rest when you are tired and get enough sleep.
- continue to work, if possible.
- stay occupied with meaningful activities.
- give both physical and emotional affection.
- practise safer sex.
- meet as often as you can with your friends and family.
- talk to someone you trust about the diagnosis and the illness.
- seek medical attention for health problems and follow the advice you are given this includes taking steps to prevent other infections. This is particularly important in infections like tuberculosis where the treatment is for a longer period of time.
- maintain personal hygiene by cleaning teeth daily, bathing daily and changing clothes. It is very important for women to keep clean during menstruation by using clean pads/cloth and keeping the genitalia clean to prevent infections of the vagina and womb
- reduce stress as much as possible. Use relaxation methods (meditation, yoga, etc.) regularly
- use appropriate herbal remedies to supplement medicines.

And you should avoid as far as possible:

- alcohol and tobacco

  Alcohol can damage the liver which can cause other problems and lower the body's immunity (defences) against illnesses. Alcohol also makes one forget some important practices like using a condom during sexual intercourse which can infect the partner with HIV and also expose one to other sexually transmitted diseases.

  Tobacco (cigarette) damages the lungs and other parts of the body and makes it easy for infection to enter.

  Both alcohol and tobacco are- expensive and the money spent on these items could be utilized for buying foods which are nutritious which will make the body strong to fight illnesses.
- other infections including further exposures to HIV; each infection you get weakens the immune system further making you susceptible to subsequent infections, which make your immune system weaker still, and so on.
- using unprescribed medicines - certain medicines can have side-effects that may be particularly harmful if you have AIDS.
- isolation - your family and friends can do a lot to help you keep active and feeling positive; do not shut them out of your life.

- using recreational drugs - like unprescribed medicines - these can be harmful.

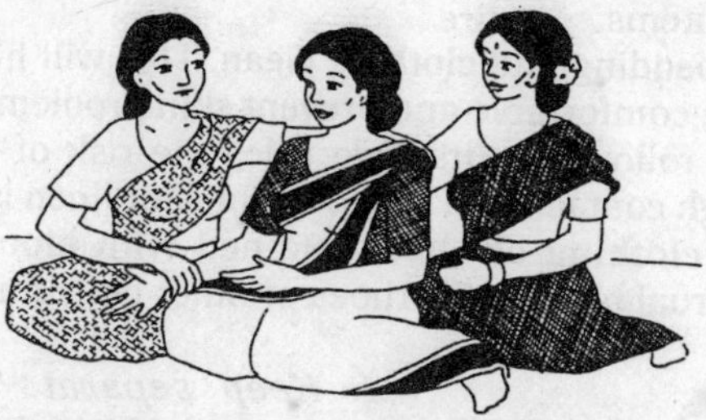

PREVENTING HIV TRANSMISSION IN THE HOME

Radha, during her visits to the homes of people with AIDS, pays great attention to two important issues. She had learned that there are two issues that are of great concern to people with AIDS and their families. The first is how to prevent HIV transmission from the person with AIDS to anyone else in the home or the community. The second is how to maintain a safe environment that does not expose the person with AIDS to unnecessary—infections.

As you learned from the first part of the story, HIV can be transmitted from one person to another. However, unlike some other infectious organisms, HIV is not easily transmitted except by unprotected sexual intercourse or close blood-to-blood contact. The virus dies quickly outside the human body.

There is no risk of acquiring HIV from people infected with it (or people with AIDS) in the home situation provided you follow certain simple rules.

Because AIDS is known to be fatal, people are concerned about whether it is safe to care for an infected person.

Those providing home care should be taught to follow these rules:

- Wash hands with soap and water after changing soiled bed sheets and clothing, and after having contact with body fluids.
- Keep wounds covered. Both care givers and people with AIDS should cover any open wounds they may have on their hands or other places likely to have contact with other people, their bedding or clothing. Cover open wounds with a bandage or cloth.
- If blood from an infected person is spilt, then it should be immediately cleaned with a disinfectant such as bleaching powder (1% solution). Household gloves (rubber gloves) should be worn and if gloves are not available, then the hands should be covered with paper or polythene bags.

Hands should always be cleaned afterwards with soap and water.

- Use a piece of plastic or paper, gloves or a big leaf to handle soiled items.
- Keep bedding and clothing clean. This will help keep sick people comfortable and prevent skin problems.
- If you follow the first two rules the risk of transmission through contact with soiled clothing or linen is very low. To clean clothing or sheets stained with blood (including menstrual blood), diarrhoea or other body fluids:

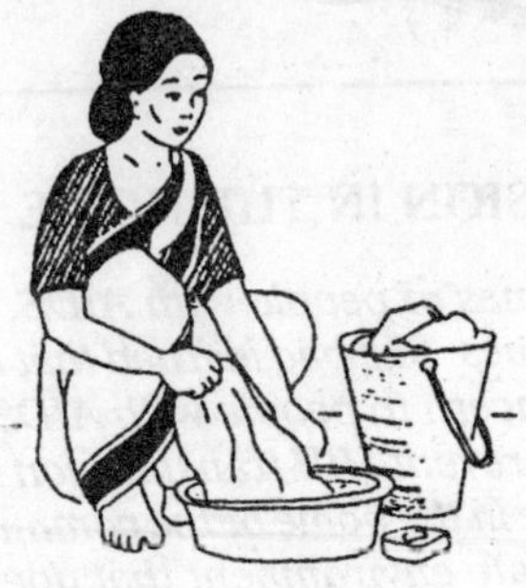

1. *Keep separate from other household laundry.*
2. *Holding an unstained part, rinse off any blood or diarrhoea with water be particularly careful if there are large amounts of blood, such as after childbirth. If possible ideally, the blood-stained clothes should be soaked in bleach solution for twenty minutes.*
3. *Wash in soapy water, hang to dry and fold or iron as you would normally.*

- Don't share sharp skin-piercing instruments. Don't share toothbrushes, razors, needles, or anything else that can cut or come into contact with blood.

It is important to emphasize that HIV *is not* spread during normal social contact People should not worry about getting other sexually transmitted diseases (STDs) like syphilis or gonorrhoea, from everyday contact with people, and they should have no greater worry regarding HIV or AIDS. However, it is important to avoid other common infections that are spread by normal social contact, such as diarrhoea.

AVOIDING RESPIRATORY INFECTIONS

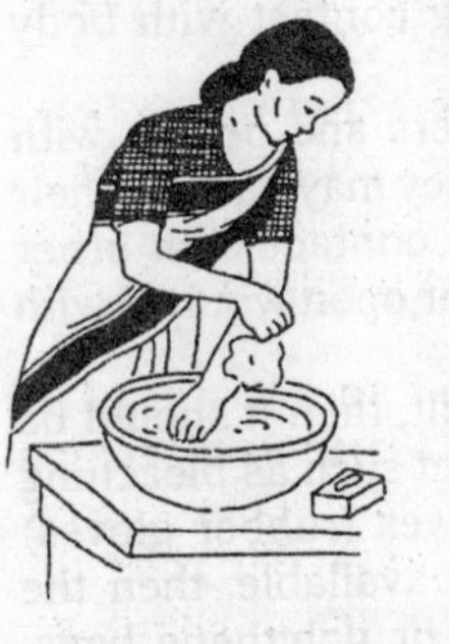

As was explained in Chapter 2, people with HIV or AIDS have a weak immune system and therefore the body's resistance to fight infections is low. Each infection they get weakens their immune system further. But there is a lot you can do to ensure that they are protected from infections of all types. Good hygiene (cleanliness) in the home is an important part of protecting against diseases such as diarrhoea and respiratory infections.

But many organisms that cause opportunistic infections already live in the body, and will cause disease if their immune system becomes too weak to stop them. Therefore, avoiding contact with healthy people is not necessary.

The following box gives tips on what people should do in their homes so that everyone in the family (including the person with AIDS) is safer from common infections.

GOOD HYGIENE

Always wash your hands before:

- cooking
- eating
- feeding another person
- giving medicine
- caring for a baby.

Always wash hands after:

- using a toilet or changing nappies
- caring for pets or animals
- working e.g., in the fields.

Other practices that ensure good hygiene:

- Washing eating utensils, including items for babies, with soap and water.
- Washing all raw fruits and vegetables with clean water. Eating freshly cooked food as far as possible.
- Keeping food covered so that flies cannot sit on it.
- Washing objects that a child or infant frequently puts in its mouth with soap and clean water.
- Storing food properly to prevent it from spoiling and causing infection.
- Getting water for drinking from a safe source.
- Storing water in a clean container, covered with a clean lid and using a ladle to take out water.
- Washing bed linen, towels and clothes with soap and water.
- Keeping the house and surroundings clean so that no flies or mosquitoes breed.
- Covering mouth when sneezing or coughing.
- Avoiding spitting or always spit into a container, not on the ground.
- Kissing babies on the top of their heads rather than on the lips.
- Disposing of waste properly by:
  - putting soiled things like nappies, used tissues and other soiled objects out of the reach of children until they can be removed from the home by putting them in a container that is hard to open until you can clean or dispose of them properly. The same should be done for household wastes too.
  - using a pit latrine, or burning or burying objects.
  - using a latrine to pass stools to avoid breeding of flies and to keep water sources safe from contamination.
- disposing waste water safely to prevent mosquitoes from breeding by using proper drainage or building soakage pits.

AVOIDING MALARIA

Malaria is a very common illness caused by an infection passed by the bite of a mosquito. Malaria weakens the body. Repeated attacks of malaria cause anaemia as it destroys the red blood cells in the body. There are many things you can do to revent this infection and, therefore, prevent the further weakening of the body.

These include:

- Use bednets (mosquito nets preferably treated with insecticide) or a sheet to protect the family when they sleep. Cover the baby's cradle or bed with a mosquito net or thin clotl .
- Use insecticide sprays and repellents to protect your home or body from any mosquitoes in the area.
- Insect proof the windows and doors by using wire net.
- Drain any standing water which may be a mosquito breeding ground in your community.

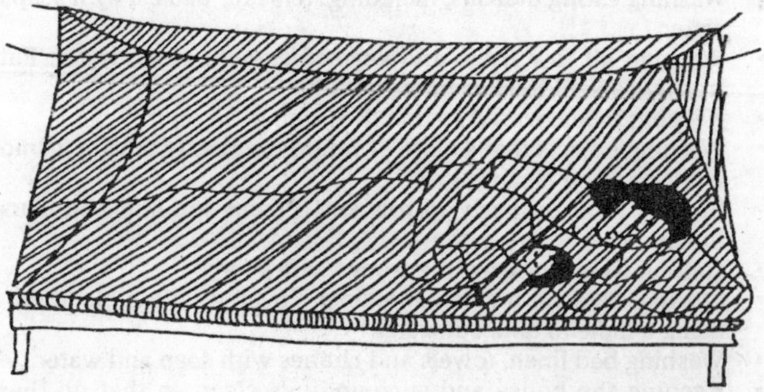

4

Women, Children and HIV

Women are sexually, economically and biologically more vulnerable to HIV infection and AIDS. The social cultural and economic impact of the epidemic on women will be greater compared to men.

This chapter continues with the third part of Story 1 which is again followed by teaching notes. The story is again presented in a way that you can use directly when teaching. The story talks about women's vulnerability to HIV, their increased burden due to caring, difficulties in negotiating safer sex and concerns about having children when HIV infected.

THE STORY CONTINUES–RADHA AND THE WOMEN

Now let us join Radha and the community group again, where we left off before. It is ...

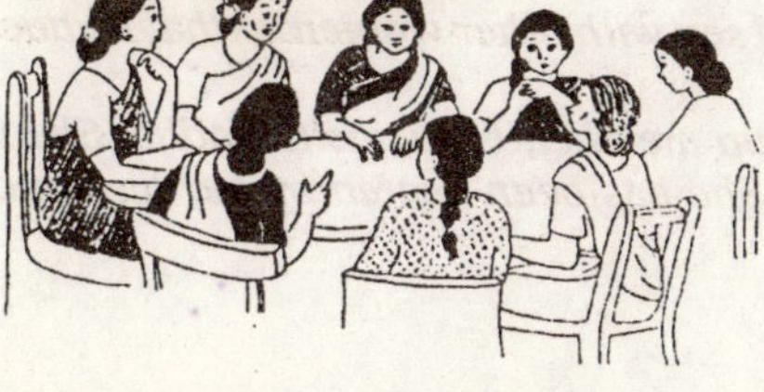

LATE 1994

More and more women join the community group. Some of these women, like Radha, have been infected with HIV. They are also care givers for their families. Others are not infected but want to be involved.

Many women whose husbands are ill due to AIDS have to work outside their homes to support their families. The women have been concerned for sometime about the work load of women as care givers and providers of needs of the family. To relieve women of some of these responsibilities, the group organized several activities. With the help of a religious group who have been providing support to the people with HIV or AIDS, care takers have been arranged for people who are very ill. The women decide to open a creche in coordination with the local authorities responsible for women and child programmes. The creche also provides some educational activities for school-going and preschool children. With the money which the community organization has earned, scholarships have been provided to school-going children. These activities decreased the burden on the women.

One day, one of the group members brings Shanti to attend the meeting. Shanti has been deserted by her husband. Shanti's story is as follows:

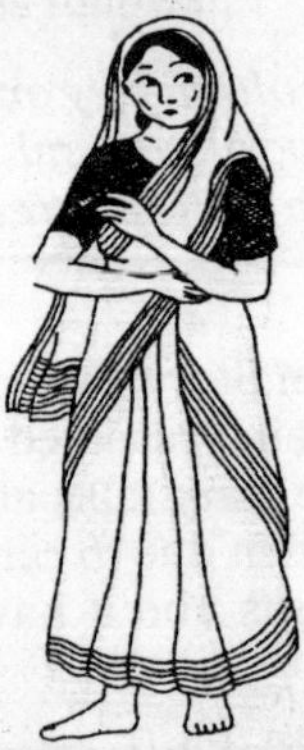

Shanti's husband works in another town and comes home for a few days only once in a month. Shanti had itching and boils around the vagina. When she went for treatment to a clinic, she was counselled and her blood was taken for testing. She was told that she is infected with HIV. When she mentioned this to her husband, he accused her of having relationships with some other man and threw her out of the house. Her husband never admitted to her about his sexual relationships with other women and that he was on treatment for boils on his penis, which he contracted during unprotected sex. Shanti has had sex only with her husband.

The women discuss Shanti's case, the vulnerability of women and how to help. They feel that they must discuss this issue in the next community meeting. With the efforts of the community group, Shanti's husband has taken her back home. He has also decided to stop having unprotected sex with other women so that he does not spread the infection.

One morning another group member, Uma, visits Radha. She is all bruised and is crying. She has been beaten by her husband. Her story is as follows:

Uma has heard about STDs and AIDS in the women's group meeting. When she finds that her husband is having a discharge from his penis, she requests him to use a condom during sex. Her husband refuses and beats Uma for refusing to have sex with him. He forces her to have sex with him. He accuses her of giving him the infection by saying that the discharge she had from her vagina is responsible for his infection.

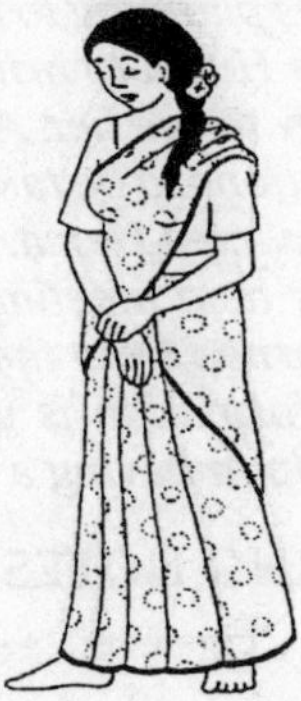

Uma is totally dependent on her husband for money, food and clothing.

Radha and the other women in the group discuss the need for Uma and other women to earn some money so that they can be in a position to decide for themselves in matters which directly concern them.

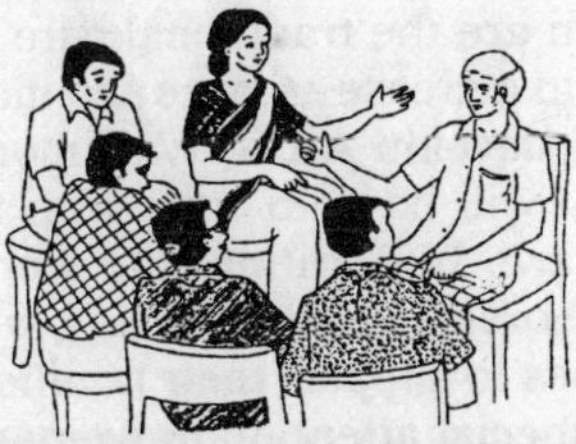

The group asked the local doctor to attend a meeting to talk to the men about HIV. Gradually the men and women were able to talk more openly and men are now helping out when someone is sick at home.

With the introduction of income-generating schemes, women are slowly earning some money and are picking up courage to play a more active role in negotiating safer sexual relationships.

It [illegible] ce Kannan died. Radha still feels sad when [illegible] he feels that if she had known earlier that [illegible] V, she would have considered all options, [illegible] n the pregnancy. Radha spends time talking to wo[illegible] are infected, about the problems and risk of pregnancy for women who are infected with HIV.

Hema is infected with HIV and is pregnant. She is fully aware of the risk to the baby and to herself but wants to continue with the pregnancy. Radha encourages her to go to the local health centre for antenatal care.

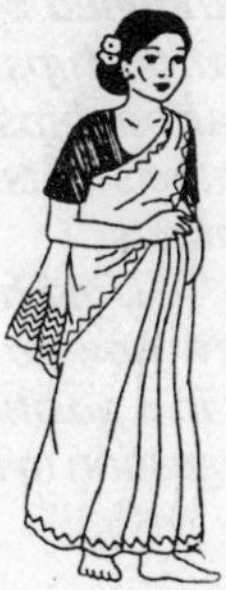

The health worker gives her advice on care during pregnancy. Hema is planning to have the delivery at home. The health worker advises Hema to bring the birth attendant who will be doing the delivery to see her. Advice on preparations for delivery and what precautions to be taken is given by the health worker. Radha also accompanies Hema.

In their next meeting, Radha shares with women the things she had learned from the health worker. She tells the women that all this information is useful for any woman who is pregnant and will help in having a safe delivery.

TEACHING NOTES ON WOMEN, CHILDREN AND HIV/AIDS

The women's group did many things to decrease the burden on women as care givers. They arranged for care of the sick so that they could go for work to support the family. A creche was arranged to take care of the children. Scholarships were given from the community funds to help children to complete their schooling.

Women as care givers

In most societies, women are the traditional care givers for their families. This role is going to increase as more and more people become infected with HIV and develop AIDS. With more women getting infected with HIV, they will have to cope with their own illnesses and the burden of care. In addition, the women have responsibilities for household chores. In many families, women will have to work outside their homes to support their families. You, as providers of care, should pay special attention to women in these families. It is important to decrease some of the burden on the women by redistributing household tasks, arranging for child care and by supporting education of children, etc. Such arrangements are important even when women do not work outside their homes. Care programmes should provide support and help families to rural areas.

Vulnerability of women

Shanti was infected with HIV by her husband, but was abandoned by him. Shanti's husband accused her of having sexual relationships with other men even though Shanti never had any relationships outside marriage. Her husband had many sexual contacts outside marriage and he got STDs and HIV through these contacts.

Uma had adequate knowledge about STDs and HIV and she knew how to protect herself against these infections. But she was not in a position to insist that her husband use a condom In fact, the suggestion to use a condom made him suspicious of her having sexual contacts outside their marriage. He forced her into having sexual intercourse with him because as his wife she was not supposed to say no. In addition, Uma's husband accused her of being responsible for the boils on his penis. Uma was dependent on her husband and so she couldn't object to her husband beating her.

Increased sexual vulnerability

Women are more vulnerable sexually because of cultural expectations. In many societies, women are not supposed to talk about sex or make decisions about sex. They do not have the right to suggest safer sexual practices, including condom use, which could protect them from HIV infection as well as other sexually transmitted diseases. Women are expected to be 'faithful' to their partners, while men having several sexual partners is often overlooked. In many societies, women generally get married to older men who are likely to have been sexually active for a longer period and therefore, more likely to have become infected. All these factors are very much linked to women's low status in society.

Increased economic vulnerability

Women are often economically dependent, a fact which takes away their freedom to negotiate safer sexual practices.

Increased biological vulnerability of women

The chances of entry of HIV into the body through the lining of the sexual organs during sex are more in women compared to men. The same trend is seen in other STDs too.

Studies in many countries have found that male-to-female transmission of HIV appears to be 2-4 times as efficient as female-to-male transmission.

STDs in women present fewer symptoms and therefore often go unnoticed and untreated. Also the chances of women reaching a facility where proper treatment for STDs is available are low. As was discussed in Chapter 2, STDs increase the chances of HIV transmission.

Vulnerability of young women and girls

Young women and girls are particularly vulnerable. For example, in many countries it is common for men to select significantly younger women as wives, making them culturally vulnerable to HIV infection at a younger age.

Their immature cervix and relatively low vaginal mucus production presents less of a barrier to HIV, making them biologically more vulnerable to infection.

Sexual abuse and child prostitution also contribute to the vulnerability of girls and young women to infection with HIV.

As a consequence, women are increasingly becoming infected with HIV at a younger age than men, and more girls and young women are becoming infected in their teens and early twenties than women in any other age group.

Increased vulnerability to transmission through blood

Women receive blood transfusions more often than men because of anaemia and complications of pregnancy and childbirth, including unsafe at ortions. Therefore, they are more vulnerable to HIV infection through untested blood.

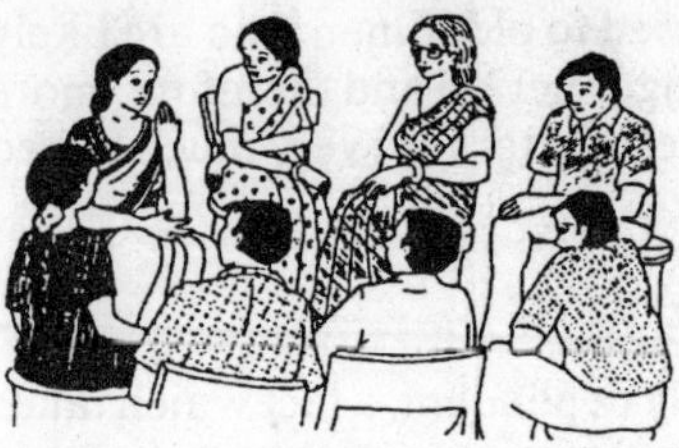

Initiality, the group Radha started had only women, but it was expanded to include men. Men in the community were consulted in the cases of Shanti and Uma. Radha learned at a very early stage in her community work that involvement of men was essential for the success of the various AIDS-related activities started by women.

To reduce the vulnerability of women to HIV infection, it is important to ensure support of men at all levels. Educational programmes must focus on responsibilities of men and women in preventing transmission by engaging in safer sex practices. Men and women should be encouraged to share care giving responsibilities and therefore, programmes for training in care should include both.

Issues concerning pregnancy

For many women, the news that they have AIDS is directly related to their role as a mother. Most women who become infected with HIV and develop AIDS do so early in their lives, during or even before the time that they bear children. This means they must face difficult choices.

Many times it is during, or immediately following, a pregnancy that a woman discovers she is infected with HIV or has AIDS. This is especially distressing news because pregnancy for a woman with HIV or AIDS brings with it the risk of having an infected child and the possibility of worsening her own illness. These painful facts are even worse in places where the status of women is influenced by their ability to bear children and where it may be socially unacceptable or very difficult to take the steps to avoid pregnancy abstinence from sexual intercourse or contraception or to consider terminating a pregnancy.

Though there are many aspects of HIV transmission during pregnancy that are not yet understood, some information is available that can help women with HIV to decide whether or not to start a pregnancy, or to prepare these women for the possible consequences of pregnancy.

If a woman is infected with HIV and becomes pregnant, the risk of her having, an HIV-infected child is approximately one in three. Some children are infected in the womb, some during delivery and some through breast-feeding.

If a woman has AIDS, she is more likely to have a complicated pregnancy, with problems during the pregnancy itself, during delivery of the baby, or after the birth.

Women with HIV infection or partners of men who are infected with HIV will need information for the following reasons:

- to help them to decide whether to become pregnant or not
- to help them to decide whether to terminate a pregnancy
- to discuss methods of contraception and other forms of fertility regulation
- to manage a pregnancy
- to plan for care of a child who is or is not infected

You can be helpful in discussing issues surrounding pregnancy and HIV and help them in making difficult decisions. In some cases you will also have to refer people for further advice from other counselling or medical services, if available.

Hema wants to continue with her pregnancy even though she knows she is infected with HIV. Radha spent a lot of time talking to her about the risks to the baby and to herself. But Hema and her husband are sure that Hema must continue with the pregnancy. Hema has been advised by the health worker about care during pregnancy and childbirth. The health worker also advised the birth attendant about special precautions.

Details of what to do at home during pregnancy and childbirth are given in Chapter 7.

Special issues concerning children with AIDS

Radha learned from personal experience and from her visits to the community that HIV infection and AIDS among children is a major worry among people. During her training, Radha was taught that there are some special points to remember while caring for children with AIDS. Radha taught the families about caring for their children which not only will benefit children with HIV/AIDS, but also other children.

Kannan was sick from birth. He had frequent attacks of diarrhoea and he did not gain any weight. His condition deteriorated and he died before his first birthday.

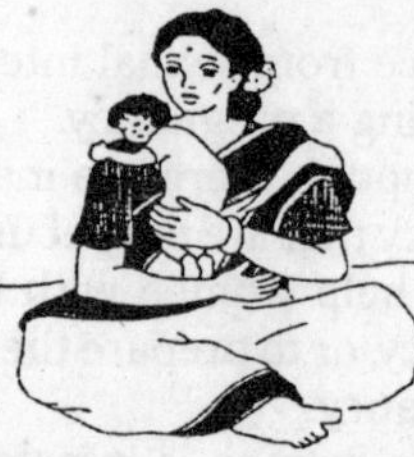

AIDS in children is very much like AIDS in adults. However, in children the disease is more difficult to diagnose correctly, and the blood test cannot be donor With certainty until the child is at least 15 months old. Small babies an children with AIDS often have fever, diarrhoea and coughing, ear and throat infections and to not gain weight properly, but these are common symptoms that may have other causes. This long period of uncertainty is very difficult for families.

Babies with HIV infection usually develop the symptoms of AIDS more quickly than adults do. This is because their immune systems are less developed and the blood not resist HIV, or fight opportunistic infections as effectively as adults.

The fact that a mother cannot know for sure, even with a test, that her-baby is infected with HIV is very distressing. Even if a child is infected there can be years of life and things that can be done to make those years as healthy and safe as possible.

Mothers and fathers need information about HIV infection and AIDS in children to help them understand the facts and then they need support to help them cope during this time of uncertainty by focusing on their child's life and health rather than on the fear of illness.

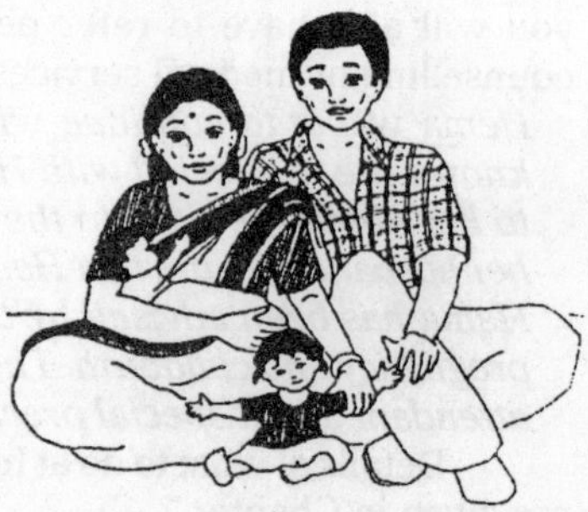

General rules on caring for a child with HIV infection or AIDS

Feed the child well

For a child less than four to six months old the best food is breast milk. Breast milk is important because it gives an infant protection against many types of infections. Also, since breast milk is clean, the infant is not at risk of getting diarrhoea as it is with milk of other types.

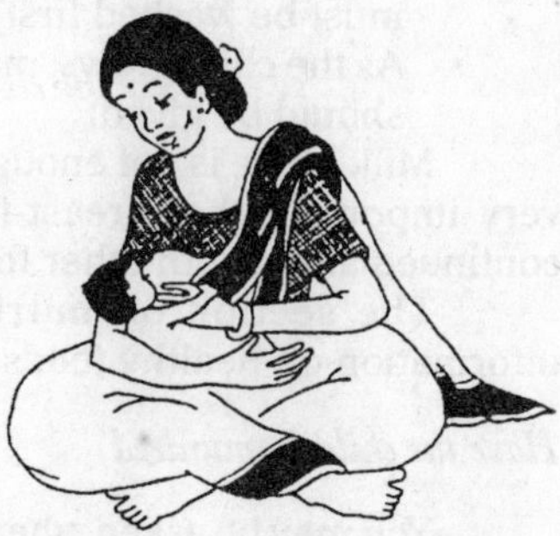

However, the fact that HIV can be passed through breast milk makes it difficult for a mother with HIV to decide what is best for the child. In many areas of the world, the risk of transmission of HIV by breast-feeding is low compared with the risk of the infant dying of other infectious diseases if not breast fed.

As the health care worker, you will have to help the HIV-infected mother weigh the possible risks to the infant of breast-feeding versus not breast-feeding, taking in to account such things as:

- whether many of the children in the area are at risk of, or die from infections and poor nutrition.
- whether there is a good alternative to breast-feeding available that is clean, safe, nutritious and affordable.

It is recommended that if the HIV-infected mother lives in a place where man, children die at a young age from infectious diseases (like respiratory infections or diarrhoea), she should breast-feed her infant, even if she is infected with HIV or has AIDS.

However, if a mother with HIV can give a clean, safe and nutritious substitute for breast-milk that is affordable for the entire period it is required, then this would be a good choice. If she decides to feed her baby using breast-milk substitutes rather than breast-milk, she must:

- use clean water, which has been boiled and then cooled, and.
- clean equipment (teats and bottles, cups and spoons) with every feed.
- be sure that when she mixes the milk substitute she uses the right amounts by following the directions carefully. She must not add more water in an effort to save money as this can lead to malnutrition in her child.

If she cannot follow all of the above requirements, all of the time, advise her to breast-feed her baby.

Once a child is four to six months old it should be given some solid foods along with the breast-milk.

- Preparations of staple foods high in energy (oils, fats and sugar are good sources of energy) should be given.
- Foods that are warm and either soft or mashed can be given

with a spoon or your fingers (don't forget utensils and hands must be washed first).

- As the child grows, more and larger quantities of adult foods should be given.

Milk alone is not enough for a child after six months, but it is very important that breast-feeding or a nutritious substitute be continued along with other foods.

The section on nutrition problems in Chapter 6 gives information on healthy foods.

Have the child immunized

You may be asked whether an infant with HIV or AIDS should be given vaccines against the common childhood illnesses. All infants including those with HIV infection and AIDS, should be given the standard vaccines against diptheria, pertussis (whooping cough) and tetanus (DPT vaccine) and against poliomyelitis (Polio) and measles. This should be done in accordance with the immunization schedules of your country. In many countries, the BCG vaccine is given to all infants at birth to prevent tuberculosis. The only exception is that if an infant has clinical symptoms of AIDS, such as failure to thrive and frequent infections, it should not receive BCC, but should receive all other vaccines.

Make sure the child gets early treatment for infections

The advice given earlier in this chapter on avoiding common infections is important. As children become older they will need to learn these things for themselves, for example about washing their hands after going to the toilet or latrine, and about the importance of washing their hands before eating. Protecting children with AIDS from other infections is more difficult than protecting adults because children tend to put things in their mouths, and they are exposed to more illnesses that are new to them.

It is much better for a family to go to the same health care setting where the child's health history is known for the process of immunization and treatment or any childhood illnesses as well as for treatment of AIDS symptoms than it is to keep changing or shopping around.

Note. Chapter 6 of this handbook describes the common symptoms of AIDS and how to treat them. Many of the symptoms children show are the same as those experienced by adults and the advice for their care is also very similar in most cases. Where the treatment of children is different, this is explained.

Treat the child as normal

Many of the infants who are infected with HIV will have

months or years of life without symptoms. Every effort should be made to help them lead as normal a life as possible. This includes letting them spend time with other children. HIV cannot he spread by the child's urine, saliva, faeces or vomit. A child with HIV cannot infect others by playing with them or sharing toys. Children should go to school as usual, except when there is an outbreak of an infection in the other children which puts the child with HIV infection at risk of becoming ill.

5

Care of the Dying

This chapter begins with the final part of the story about the family you first met in Chapter 2. Radha is dead now and her mother Prema tells how she died and how her community reacted.

The rest of the chapter provides information you need to give to family members who are caring for someone who is dying from AIDS. The information is presented in a way that you can use when speaking directly to the family.

THE LAST PART OF THE STORY–RADHA'S LEGACY

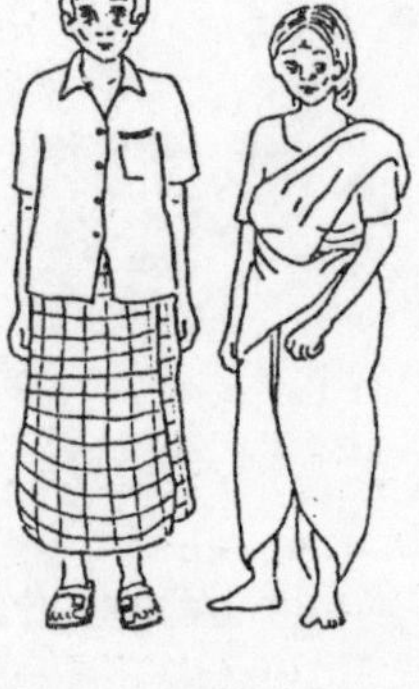

EARLY 1995

Radha died last night. I am Prema, Radha's mother. Her father, Raman, and I will miss her. Our family and community have lost another young person. But we all must die in our time and it was her time. She went as one should, proud and in peace. She taught us in her death much about our lives. Let me tell you of her dying, it was good and perhaps we shall all live and die so well.

She was carrying this infection, who knows for how long. It seems to come from nowhere. I am told that so many of our young people already have the infection.

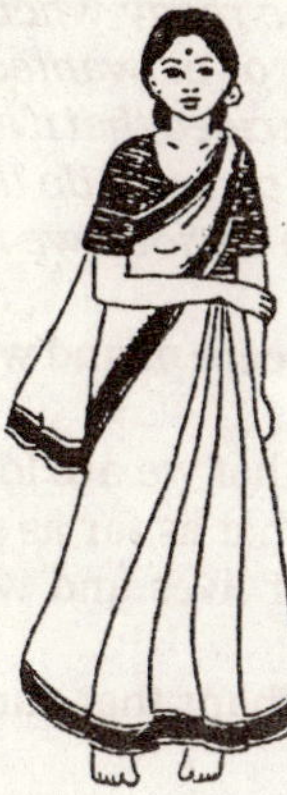

Radha lost her husband two years back and a child before that. Then she got her blood test done. She told us about her infection and that Ravi and Kannan both had died of AIDS. She told us that there was just a bit more time before she too would go. We decided that we must go to Radha and help support her. Radha decided that she has to fight the infection for her own sake and for her little Meenakshi. She was so sure that it was up to us to teach and keep our little ones free of this illness until they could learn to keep themselves free.

Radha wanted to help other people with HIV infection or AIDS. So she took special training to counsel and care for sick people.

Long before her death Radha said it was important to do things before she died and to plan for these. We began to sit together, many of us. At first it included only women - women who were sick or widowed, had lost their children or were worried.

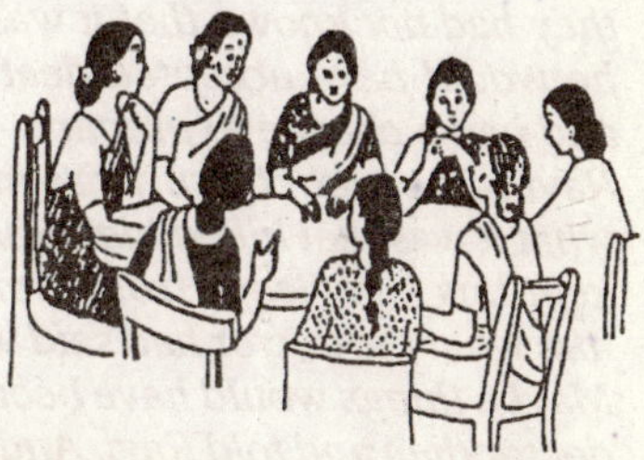

We had seen people die alone with no family or friends near them. We remember the young man in our area who, before his death, had instructed his brothers to give his share of the property to his wife and children. But his wishes were ignored and his wife and children were thrown out of their home. We know of people who die rejected, people die without names or a family to remember them. It was too much sorrow for us all to bear. "Not us, not me', we each said.

Most of us have learnt or thought of death only in our religion. We don't talk of it anywhere else in our lives. Earning money, raising children, seeing that they are educated, building the future are what we know best. How strange death seems when we look it in the face how little related to our lives and how difficult to talk about. Radha had great courage to speak of this.

Radha said that each person needed to make a plan for "living and dying proud" as she called it, so that even when death seemed very far away we could be sure we would be ready when it was our time to die. We talked about what each of us wanted at the end that would make death not so bitter. We decided that if a person can do things to have a "good life" then they can also do things to have a "good death" These are the things we decided we must be sure of in order to meet and accept death:

- that those we care about will be taken care of and will try to accept our leaving them.
- that we are not alone in our fear and that we are loved.
- that our wishes will be respected, so that as far as possible we shall be given full choice over our lives and what will happen to us until the end.
- that we should not be forgotten, or perhaps that our life has a meaning larger than we can know.

We began by looking at each of these things and thinking about what it would take to make them possible. Some of these are things that can happen only if all of us encourage and help each other. Within each of us the first thing we had to find was acceptance. It is in acceptance that caring can grow.

Radha always said she was sorry that when her husband died they had not known that it was because of AIDS. She is sure that he would have accepted death more easily had he known that and had a chance to prepare.

Ravi was caught by surprise in some ways and never understood what it was that killed him. She was sorry because she knows she kept this knowledge from him by her denial, and she did not tell him what the doctor had said when she took the baby to the clinic. Maybe things would have been different if she had listened to the doctor then and told Ravi. And, she knows he never meant to pass this illness to her. But, she said through not blaming anybody, not blaming herself for perhaps taking from Ravi the chance to live longer and to die in knowledge, and not blaming him for bringing this illness into their little family, because of which she lost her child - comes acceptance.

From this acceptance, she said, her heart could look outwards to give more and to ask more of the community.

Our little group of women were joined by men and then we invited the local leader. Radha wanted to start many activities which would provide care to those with AIDS and their families. But none of us knew how to plan. So, Radha contacted the people who had trained her and with their help she planned various activities.

The face of our community changed. It became a friendlier place in which to live and die. This Radha offered to us all and to herself Last night was her time and she died as she lived: an example for us all Let me tell you what she did in those last days.

Meenakshi is ten years old now. Radha had her tested at the clinic to show us and herself that caring for each other, staying together and being a family, carried no risk. Meenakshi has no HIE Radha turned the illness into the enemy, not those with the illness. Maybe now we know this enemy a little better and how to keep it away. She turned her anger at the illness into a force in all our lives.

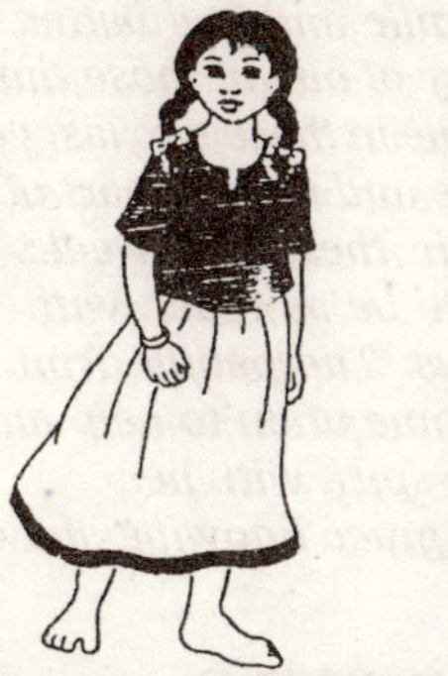

But one day, it seemed, she knew that death was near and that it could no longer be kept away. She changed. She became quieter. I argued with her then saying "Fight, fight more, it doesn't have to win now" But she said "Yes, mother, the time is short. Just as we have a time to fight and to live, so we have a time to die and mine is near. Be with me" Over these two weeks, her father and I stayed close to her as she had done for so many others.

She made it clear how Meenakshi was to be brought up and with whom she would live. The money and possessions that they had were taken into account and agreements were made on how they should be passed to others, and within her family. We did this as a community to be sure that all would honour her wishes and protect her daughter. She had seen too many others lose even this last peace.

She asked to be part of our lives even to the end. We put her bed in the centre of the main room I and the neighbours took turns telling stories, remembering the past, praying and doing what needs to be done.

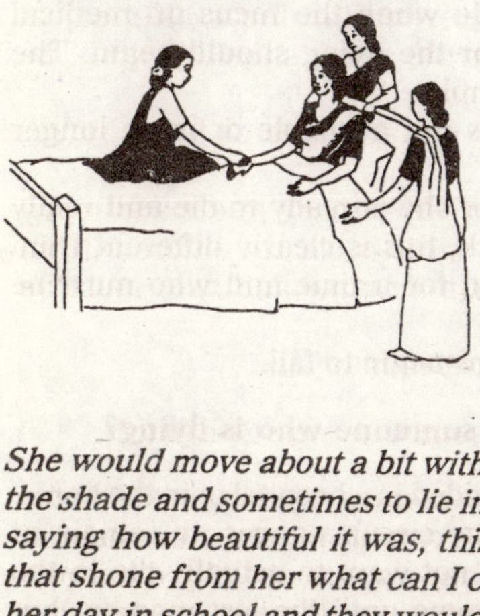

Radha had pain. It made her feel better to have her skin rubbed with oil. She said it eased the aching. The doctor had given some medicine for her pain which she would ask for sometimes but she would also say, "Amma (Mother), tell me a story or sing me a song it's better than those pills"

She would move about a bit with our help, sometimes to a bench in the shade and sometimes to lie in the breeze near the door. She kept saying how beautiful it was, this life, this earth. It was something that shone from her what can I call it's Meenakshi would tell her of her day in school and they would talk together quietly sometimes. It is hard for a girl so young who loved her mother.

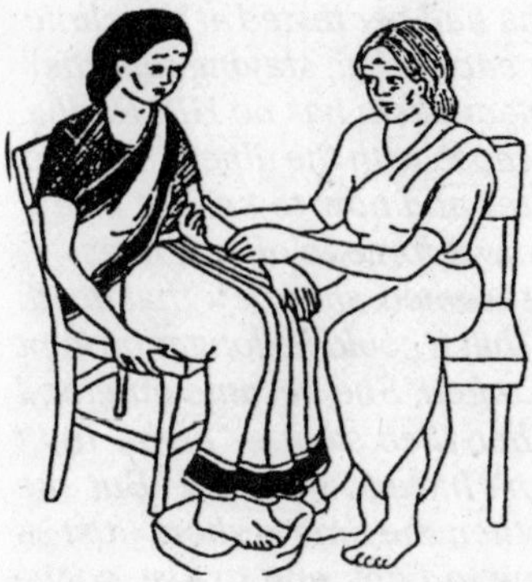

I did what she had done for so many others, reminded people of the good things they had done and helped them forget their sorrow or pain. I'd ask her, 'What did you do here on this earth that made one person smile and feel better. Tell me a story of one of those times" The temple in these two last years was more and more a part of her life and in these last weeks she seemed to be as much with God as with us. The people from the temple came often to help and to share the spirit with her.

I have lost much but I know she died in grace knowing she was loved. I hope to die so well.

TEACHING NOTES ON CARE OF THE DYING

At some point in the disease process of AIDS, there is nothing more that can be done to effectively treat the opportunistic infections, or completely relieve the symptoms that they cause. The infections or illnesses have progressed beyond what medicines can cure. At this point, the goal of all care (medical, nursing, religious and psychological) is to keep the person as comfortable as possible and to maintain their dignity. In some places this is called palliative care.

When does this time begin?

It is often difficult to decide when the focus on medical treatment should stop and care for the dying should begin. The change in care may begin, for example:

- when medical treatment is not available or is no longer effective.
- when the person says he or she is ready to die and really does appear to be very sick; this is clearly different from someone who is depressed for a time and who must be encouraged not to give up.
- when the body's vital organs begin to fail.

Where can you provide care for someone who is dying?

Care for the dying can be provided in a hospital or in the home. Most people prefer or are forced by circumstances, to remain at home. However, some people may not want to actually die in the home. They may want to stay at home until the last moment but either because of their own or the family's wishes they may want to go to the hospital to die. If this is the case, a plan for transporting them will need to be thought out.

What are the goals of caring for someone who is dying?

- keeping them comfortable and protecting them from problems that can make them feel worse.
- helping them to be as independent as possible.
- assisting them in grieving for, and coping with, the continuing losses they experience.
- helping them and their families prepare for death: this may include making a will, tending to relationships in the family or the community, and arranging for the transfer of responsibilities.
- keeping them within the community and family groups for as long as possible: family members can bring them into this part of their lives even when it seems they are too ill to enjoy or understand what is going on.

What can you do to meet these goals?

Give comfort

If the person is in constant pain, make sure that pain medication is available in regular doses. It should not be taken just when the pain is really bad.

Use relaxation techniques, such as encouraging deep breathing, or giving back rubs or body massages.

Continue basic physical care to keep the person clean and dry and to prevent skin problems, and stiffness of joints.

Encourage communication within the family and community. People with AIDS and those they love need to feel that they are not outside the love and life of their community. Help them use this time as a chance to heal old wounds and to make peace with each other. This will help to increase the comfort and acceptance of the whole family.

Provide physical contact by touching, holding hands and hugging.

Provide or arrange for counselling if desired, for example from religious representatives. They can be very helpful for spiritual counselling.

Allow the sick person independence

Accept the person's own decisions such as a refusal to eat or get up, or even a demand to get up when you think that resting would be better for them.

Respect requests, for example regarding not wanting to see visitors.

Ask them what they are feeling. Listen and allow the person to talk about how they feel.

Accept the person's feelings of anger, fear, grief and other emotions.

Prepare for death

Talk about death if the person wishes to. Many people feel that it is not good to talk about the fact that someone is going to die, as if mentioning death is a wish for death. But by discussing death openly, those around are helping the dying person to prepare for death. It may take great courage to talk about it but it can be a big help for the person to feel that their concerns are heard, that their wishes will be followed and that they are not alone. To avoid talking about death is a form of denial.

One of the most common worries is for the future of the children in a family. People may fear that their children will be hungry or lack money for school fees after they have died. Begin planning with relatives, friends or orphan programmes for the future of the children. It will ease such worries if the person knows that suitable arrangements have already been made.

The person may be worried about being in pain as he or she nears death. The fear can be lessened by knowing what it will be like. If the person asks, describe what might happen, such as difficulty in breathing, or passing in and out of consciousness. If pain medications are available, reassure the person that they will be used in order to prevent unnecessary pain.

The person may be worried about what will happen after they die. The anxiety can be lessened by helping them to write a will, by planning and writing down details such as funeral arrangements and discussing spiritual beliefs, perhaps with a representative of the person's religion.

What precautions do you or the family need to take with the body of someone who has died of AIDS?

Immediately after death, you need to follow the same rules in dealing with the body as you did when helping the person through his illness. Hands should be protected when cleaning and laying out the body, particularly if there are body fluids such as diarrhoea or blood, and then washed with soap and water afterwards. Wounds on hands or arms should be covered with a plaster or bandage.

Shortly after the person has died the virus will also die. HIV can only live and reproduce inside a living person. Therefore you do not need to worry about special precautions during the funeral itself.

The person can be either buried or cremated according to local custom.

How can you help the family after the death?

Immediately after a person has died, the family may need help to grieve or to arrange practical matters. You can offer this by listening to them. You can also assist them with the funeral arrangements in accordance with the customs and regulations of the area in which you live. Again it may be appropriate for the instructions to be written down, so none are forgotten.

The death may continue to cause practical difficulties for the family. This is particularly true if planning for the death was not done properly. Also, the family and loved ones will continue to grieve for many months. Any care or practical help you can give during this time can be useful. Setting aside time to visit and asking how they are doing will help them to think of life beyond this painful time.

6

Management of Common AIDS Symptoms in the Home

This chapter covers the management of the most common symptoms that people with AIDS are likely to develop. It provides the information which you as a health care worker or care provider need to give to people with AIDS and their families so that they can prevent and treat these symptoms at home and know when they should seek help.

Each group of health problems or symptoms is discussed under the following headings:

Problems and possible causes.

This section gives a brief description of the health problem or symptom, and how it relates to someone with AIDS. In addition, some possible reasons for the symptoms are given in order to help people think how to prevent or reduce them.

What to do at home

This section describes what people can do in the home to prevent and treat the symptoms.

Only the most simple, inexpensive and readily available medicines that may be used safely in the home are described in detail. Chapter 8 covers the use of such medicines in more detail. If available, the national standards of your country for treating specific problems should be followed; the information provided here is merely a guide.

For medicines or treatments not described here, it is the responsibility of the health care worker prescribing or distributing them to give full instructions on how and when they should be used.

This section includes home remedies for some of the

conditions. These have been taken from, "Where There is No Doctor" by Werner. D.

When sick people and their families must seek help

This section describes the symptoms and changes that should warn the person with AIDS or the family to seek help from a health care worker.. You, the health care worker, must explain to sick people and their families that the appearance of the symptoms and signs described in this section means that they need to seek the advice and help of a health care worker, preferably the health care worker they usually see, who may be working in the community, at a clinic, health centre or hospital. It is much better for people to go to the same place and work with the same health care worker repeatedly during the process of treating AIDS symptoms than keep changing or shopping around. Meeting more health care workers does not mean increasing the chances of having good health.

Notes

This section is for any notes you may have on the topic, based on your experience of treatments, on your knowledge of local conditions or on further training you may receive.

FEVER

Problems and possible causes

When a persons body temperature is too high, they have a fever. Fever is not a disease in itself but a sign that something is wrong in the body. Fever may indicate one of many different illnesses.

High fever can be dangerous, especially in small children. Fever as a symptom can make anyone feel very uncomfortable.

In people with AIDS, fevers often come and go. It is difficult to know whether the fever is a symptom of a treatable infection or whether it is due to the HIV infection itself. The causes of fever include:

- AIDS-related opportunistic infections such as tuberculosis
- endemic diseases, such as malaria
- HIV infection itself.

It is important to identify tuberculosis as early as possible because it can be easily spread to others in the home, especially to children. See Chapter 7 for more information about tuberculosis.

What to do at home

The best way to check whether someone has a fever is to use a thermometer and measure their temperature.

If you do not have a thermometer you can still get an idea of whether someone has a fever by putting the back of your hand on their forehead and the back of your other hand on your forehead. If they have a fever, you should be able to feel the difference. Their forehead will feel warmer than yours.

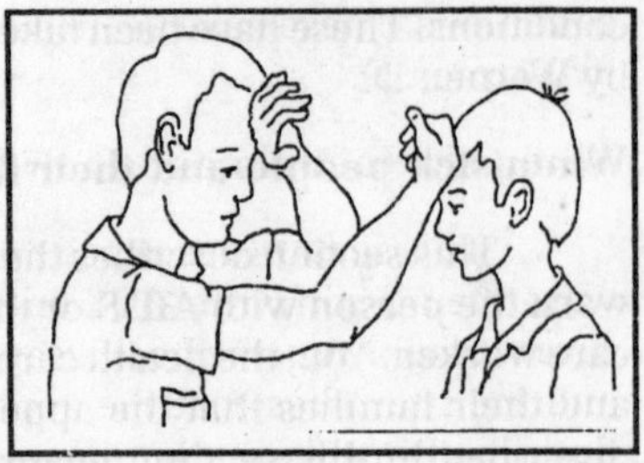

How to lower a fever

Remove any unnecessary clothing and blankets; fresh air (for example from a breeze) is not harmful and helps to lower the fever.

Cool the skin by taking baths or pouring water on it, putting cloths soaked in tepid water on the chest and forehead and fanning the cloths, or just wiping the skin with wet cloths and letting the water evaporate.

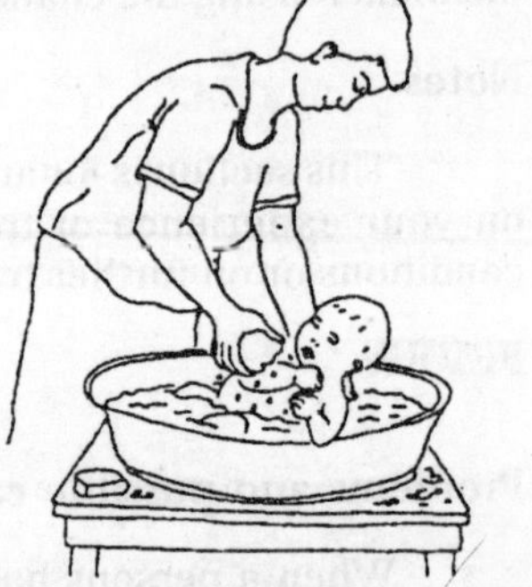

Provide plenty of water, milk tea, both or juice. When someone has a fever they lose more fluids than usual and this can make them feel worse, and can cause them to become dehydrated.

Use medicines that reduce fever (antipyretics): for example, aspirin or paracetamol, every eight hours. For children the dose is lower and depends on size (weight) or age. See Chapter Eight for specific information about these medicines.

How to manage the discomfort of fever

In between bathing and cooling the skin to lower the fever, keep the skin clean and dry.

Use lotions or powders to prevent skin problems such as rashes, sores, sore areas or broken areas.

When sick people and their families must seek help

You should encourage people to seek help if they have a fever and:

- are very hot, indicating a very high fever
- are high with chills (feeling cold) and rigors (shivers)
- the fever continues for a long time
- the fever is accompanied by coughing and weight loss
- the fever is accompanied by symptoms such as stiff neck, severe pain, confusion, unconsciousness, yellow colour in the eyes, sudden severe diarrhoea or convulsions
- are pregnant or have recently had a baby
- live in an area where malaria is common and the fever has not gone away after one treatment with antimalarial medicine; discourage people from treating themselves repeatedly with such medicine
- young infant with fever.

NOTES

DIARRHOEA

Problems and possible causes

Diarrhoea is very common in people with AIDS. The stools are usually clear and watery and are sometimes accompanied by abdominal cramps and vomiting.

What is diarrhoea?

The number of stools normally passed in a day varies with diet and age. In diarrhoea, the stools contain more water than normal - they are called loose or watery stools. They may also contain blood, in which case the diarrhoea is called dysentery. Frequent passing of normal stools is not diarrhoea.

People usually know when they have diarrhoea-the stools smell strongly or pass noisily, as well as being loose and watery. A person has diarrhoea if he passes three or more loose or watery stools in a day.

There are two types of diarrhoea, acute diarrhoea and persistent diarrhoea.

- Acute diarrhoea lasts for less than two weeks.
- Persistent diarrhoea is when someone has more than three liquid stools a day every day for more than two weeks.

The most common causes of diarrhoea in people with HIV infection are:

- intestinal infections from food or water that is not clean and fresh.
- opportunistic infections related to AIDS or side-effects of some medicines.

Why is diarrhoea dangerous?

The two main dangers of diarrhoea are dehydration and malnutrition. Dehydration is caused by the loss of large amounts of water and salt from the body, which if not treated can cause death.

How does diarrhoea cause dehydration?

The body regulates the amount of water and salts it needs by a two-way process. It takes in water and salts from the food and drink consumed. It also gets rid of excess water and salts through the stools, urine and sweat. In a healthy person there is a balance between intake and output of fluids and salts. When someone has diarrhoea, however, the intestines do not work normally and this balance breaks down. Increased amounts of water and salts are passed into the intestines and the output of water and salts becomes greater than the intake. This results in dehydration. The greater the frequency of diarrhoea the more water and salts are lost. Dehydration can also be caused by vomiting, which often accompanies diarrhoea.

Dehydration occurs faster in infants and young children, in hot climates, and in people who have fever.

How does diarrhoea cause malnutrition?

Diarrhoea (either acute or persistent) can cause malnutrition or make it worse because:

- nutrients are lost from the body in the stools,
- people with diarrhoea often do not feel hungry
- some think wrongly that they should not eat when they have diarrhoea or even for some days after the diarrhoea lessens.

What to do at home

How to prevent diarrhoea

Drink clean water

- In some areas water from sources like a tubewell, piped water supply or a handpump with an intact surrounding platform may be safe to drink. Water from ponds, rivers and lakes is not safe. To be certain that water is safe to drink, it should be strained using a clean cloth and boiled for 20 minutes to kill all the germs. Water sources should be protected from animals. Latrines should be built at a distance of at least 10 metres away from the source of water. Clothes should not be washed or one should not bathe near the sources of water.
- Water should be collected and stored in a clean, covered container and a clean long-handled ladle should be used to draw water from the container.
- Use clean drinking water when brushing your teeth.

Eat clean, safe food

- Have freshly prepared foods.
- Make sure that raw foods are washed and that cooked food, especially meat, has been cooked properly. Do not eat raw meat or fish.
- Badly washed food, or food not protected against dirt, flies and animals can be unsafe to eat because it can become contaminated with disease-causing organisms.
- If previously cooked foods are to be eaten, make sure they

have been stored safely and reheated thoroughly at a high temperature.

Wash your hands

This is particularly important. People should always wash their hands with soap and water:

- after using the latrine and after helping somebody else use the latrine and after cleaning soiled children or sick people
- before preparing food or drink for themselves or other people and before eating a after touching animals.

Use a latrine to pass stools

If no latrine is available never pass stools near a water source. Stools should be passed at least 10 metres away from the source of water supply and the stools should be covered with dirt to avoid breeding of flies.

In young children

- Breast-feed (exclusively) for the first four to six months
- Start weaning after four to six months to foods that are clean and nutritious and adequate in quantity.

Three rules for treating diarrhoea in the home

The treatment recommended here is suitable for anyone with diarrhoea, with or without AIDS.

1. Drink more fluids than usual

Dehydration can usually be prevented in the home by drinking more fluids as soon as the diarrhoea starts.

What fluids?

People should be advised by health care workers on the type of fluids to drink. It is preferable to give food-based fluids which are available at home and which normally contain some salt. These will replace the water and salts lost in diarrhoea. Examples are: rice water (salted), salted butter milk, vegetable or chicken soup with salt. Examples of other suitable fluids are plain clean water, green coconut water; and unsweetened fresh fruit juice.

Fluids that should be avoided are sweetened fruit drinks, sweetened tea, most commercial soft drinks, coffee and some medicinal teas. Drinks sweetened with sugar draw water out of the body and worsen the diarrhoea and dehydration.

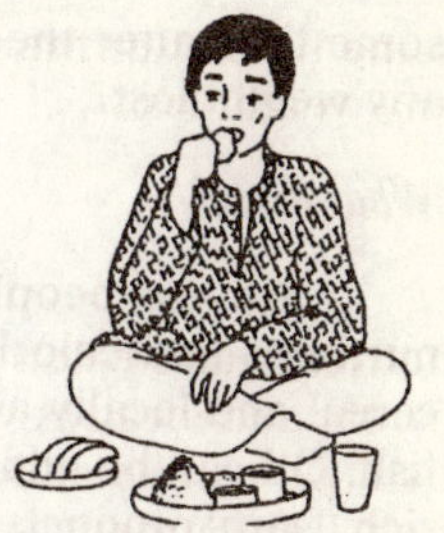

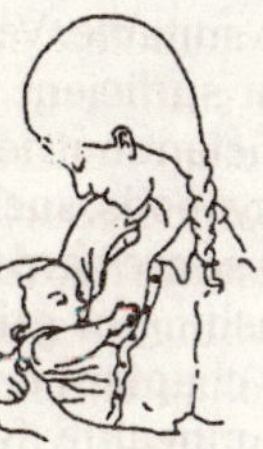

In the case of breast-fed infants with diarrhoea, the mother should continue to breast-feed and try to give feeds more often than normal (at least every three hours).

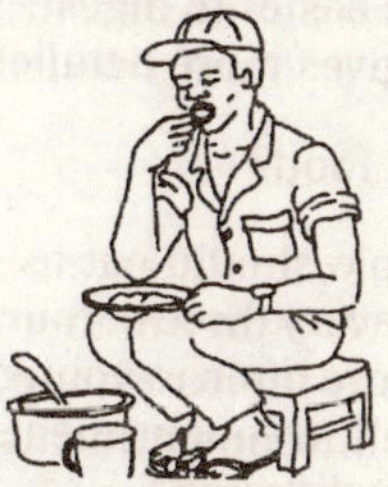

How much fluid?

Drink as much as possible

If someone does not feel thirsty they may have to force themselves to drink. It may help people to keep a glass of water nearby and sip some of it every five to ten minutes.

It is particularly important to encourage childre with diarrhoea to drink. Give children under two years old about a quarter to a half of a large cupful of fluid (50-100 milliliters) after each loose stool. Give older children one half to one large cupful (100-200 milliiliters) after each loose stool.

2. Continue to eat

If people lose their appetite when they have diarrhoea this can cause malnutrition or make existing malnutrition worse, and will not decrease the diarrhoea. The fluids taken in lo not replace the need for food. It is very important for people to take the nutrients needed to stay strong and prevent weight loss - a strong person will resist illness better.

Even if someone does not feel hungry they should eat small amounts of nutritious and easily digestible food frequently. After the diarrhoea has stopped, an extra meal every day for two weeks will help to regain any weight lost during the illness.

It is particularly important to encourage young children with diarrhoea to eat. Some children will continue to need extra food for some time after the diarrhoea has gone to make sure they regain any weight lost.

What foods?

Advise people to eat foods with the largest amounts of nutrients and calories relative to bulk. These should be mixes of cereal and locally available beans, or mixes of cereal and meat or fish. Oil can be added to these foods to make them more energy-rich. Dairy products, eggs and bananas are also suitable. Very dilute soups are recommended as fluids, but are not sufficient as foods because they fill you up without providing sufficient nutrients.

Advise people to avoid high-fibre or bulky foods, such as fruit and vegetable peels, and whole-grain cereals; these are hard to digest.

Prepare foods by cooking well, and mashing or grinding to make them easier to digest. The section in this chapter on nutrition problems gives more detailed information about healthy foods.

How much food?

People should eat as much as they want. They should take some food every three or four hours (six times each day) - food should be given more often to young children with diarrhoea. A person may prefer small, frequent meals and these are best because they are more easily digested.

3. Recognize and treat dehydration early

People should watch for signs of dehydration which are as follows:

- feeling thirsty
- feeling irritable or lazy
- skin going back slowly when pinched

People with these signs should take oral rehydration solution (ORS) used by health care workers to treat people with dehydration, and it can also be used in the home. It is made by dissolving a packet of ORS in clean drinking water. It would be best if cooled water that has previously been boiled could be used.

ORS packets are available in most parts of the world. Dissolve the contents of the packet in the amount of water indicated on the

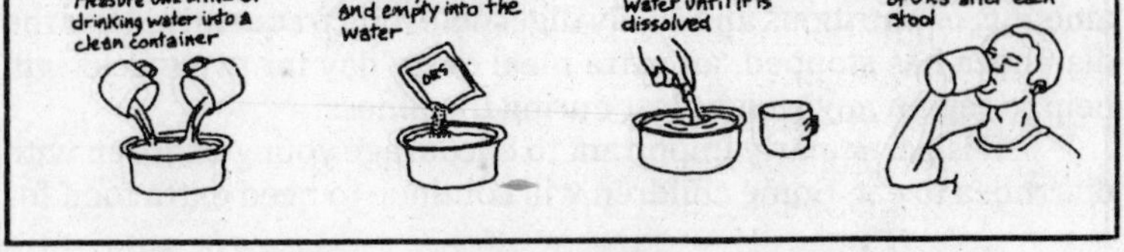
Measure ONE LITRE of drinking water into a clean container
Open the packet of Oral Rehydration Salts and empty into the water
ORS
Stir the ORS and water until it is dissolved
Drink one cup full of ORS after each stool

packet. Not all packets are of the same size so people will have to read the instructions to be sure how much water to add. If they use too little water, the drink could make the diarrhoea worse. If they use too much water, the drink will be less effective. A packet making up a litre of solution is to be prepared as shown below in the pictures.

The mixture should be stirred well and kept covered after use. The left-over solution should be thrown out after 24 hours.

Other treatments for diarrhoea

Discourage the use of medicines at home to control diarrhoea. Further details about when to use such medicines are given in the section on medicines for diarrhoea in Chapter 8.

For severe stomach cramps that sometimes accompany diarrhoea, paracetamol may be helpful. Recommendations on the dose to take are given in the section on medicines for pain in Chapter 8.

Other problems that may come with diarrhoea

Skin irritation in the rectal area

To prevent or treat sore or broken skin you should advise the sick person to:

- clean the rectal area gently with clean water after each bowel movement and pat dry
- apply a lotion/ vaseline to help relieve the discomfort and protect the skin
- sit in warm water containing a little pinch of salt three or four times a day; this may also relieve the discomfort.

Haemorrhoids (piles)

Haemorrhoids can develop after the diarrhoea has been present for some time. The are caused by a weakening of the walls and blood vessels of the rectum. The tissue around the anus become very sore and itchy. The blood vessels may become very tender and may bleed-small amounts of blood may be noticed in stools or while cleaning the rectal area.

- Trying to relax during bowel movements and not straining or pushing too hard to pass the stools can prevent haemorrhoids.
- Sitting in a bath filled with water may help to ease the discomfort and paracetamol can be taken to relieve the pain.
- If the haemorrhoids come out of the rectum during bowel movements, pushing them back in again during cleaning can be helpful.

To help someone with diarrhoea who cannot get out of bed

Use a bedpan or other suitable plastic or metal container. Be sure it is not too high and can be used by slipping it under the person in bed. Empty the contents frequently. Do not use this container for any other purpose once it has been used as a bedpan (Change wet or soiled bedding immediately to prevent damage to the skin.

The soiled cloths must be kept separate from other household laundry. By holding the unstained part of the cloth, rinse out the stains from diarrhoea and wash it with soap and water. Dry it in the sun.

When sick people and their families must seek help

People are at risk of dehydration and should seek help if they have diarrhoea and:

- are very thirsty
- have a fever
- cannot cat or drink properly
- do not seem to be getting better
- pass many watery stools
- see blood in the stools
- have diarrhoea for more than 14 days
- are vomiting and cannot keep down fluids.

Help should be sought quickly if signs of dehydration have already developed, such as:

- the person is extremely thirsty
- the person is in an irritable or lethargic state
- the skin returns slowly after pinching in children with diarrhoea, if ORS does not alleviate diarrhoea and/or stool volume increases with ORS.

NOTES ON DIARRHOEA

SKIN PROBLEMS

Problems and possible causes

The following skin problems are common in people with AIDS and unfortunately tend to be chronic. They can be controlled with the right treatment, but rarely completely cured.

- rashes
- itching skin
- painful sores on the skin
- increased dryness of the skin
- slow healing of wounds
- boils and abscesses.

The most common causes of some of these problems include:

- yeast infections (thrush, candidiasis)
- other fungal infections (e.g. ringworm)
- bacterial infections
- shingles (herpes zoster)
- infected scabies
- poor hygiene
- allergic reactions to medicines or skin irritants
- bed sores (caused by lying in one position in bed)
- eczema
- Kaposi sarcoma.

What to do at home

As a general rule, cleaning the skin frequently with soap and clean water and keeping it dry between washing will prevent the most common problems.

Almost all skin problems involve the sensation of itching. Scratching the itching skin with fingernails can make things worse, either by breaking the skin or by introducing or spreading infection. This can be avoided by keeping nails short. Try to encourage people not to scratch any type of skin lesion or sore. However, rubbing with the flat of the fingers or gentle slapping can give some relief.

Itching can be reduced in a number of ways, including the following:

- cooling the skin with water or fanning it
- applying lotions such as calamine that are soothing and prevent the skin from becoming too dry
- not letting the skin get hot and not applying warmth to itching areas
- using home remedies, eg., boil broken wheat in water and cool the mixture. Strain the mixture and the strained fluid

can be applied on the affected areas. Starch can be used instead of wheat.

- using safe effective traditional remedies that are available locally from a herbalist.

If people have trouble with very dry skin, they may have to avoid soaps and detergents and use bath oils and skin creams as much as possible. Vaseline, glyecrine and vegetable or plant oils can be as effective as the more expensive oils and creams sold in the shops.

To prevent babies or people who are confused from scratching themselves, Cut their fingernails very short or put gloves or socks over their hands.

For children in nappies who have diarrhoea or yeast infections, the buttocks area will need special care. For example, people should:

- leave the babies bottom exposed to air as much as possible
- soak the babys bottom with warm water between nappy changes
- not let the child remain in wet nappies or cloths but remove or change them as soon as they become soiled
- avoid wiping the buttocks area; instead squeeze water from a wash cloth or pour water over the area and then pat dry
- use simple lotions provided by a health care worker or pharmacist - this may help cure rashes in the nappy area, particularly if they are treated early
- not forget to wash their hands afterwards.

Treatment of wounds

Wounds (including open sores and ulcers) which are not infected:

- Wash the affected areas with clean water - preferably water which has been boiled and cooled - mixed with a little salt (one teaspoonful of salt to one litre of clean water) or gentian violet solution (one teaspoonful of gentian violet crystals in half a litre of clean water).
- Protect by covering with clean gauze bandages or cloth, wrapped loosely.
- Put warm compresses of weak salt water on the area four times a day. Use the warm compresses as explained below.
  — Boil water with salt (one teaspoonful of salt to one litre of clean water) and allow it to cool until you can just hold your hand in it.

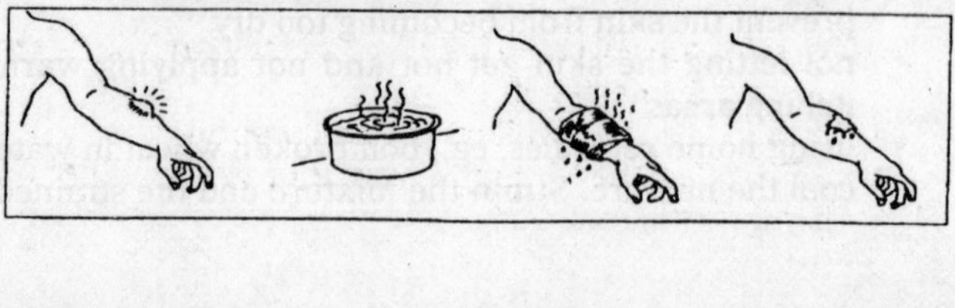

— Fold a clean cloth so that it is slightly larger than the area to be treated. Wet the cloth in the hot water and squeeze out the extra water.
— Put the cloth over the affected skin.
— Cover the cloth with a sheet of thin plastic.
— Keep the affected part raised.
— When the cloth starts to cool, put the cloth back in the hot water and repeat the process.

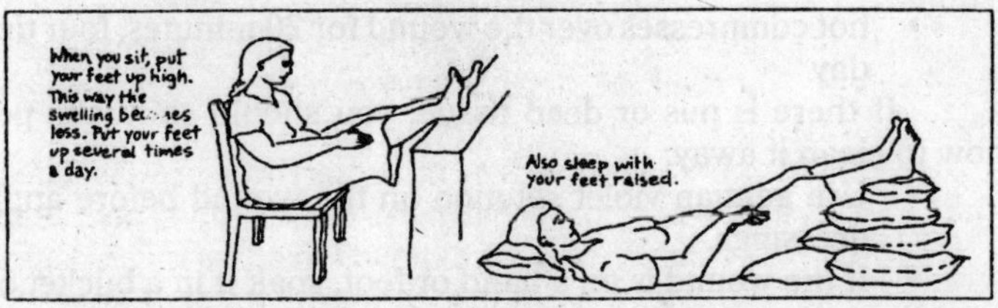

— If the wound is on the legs or feet, raise the affected area as high and as often as possible. During sleep it should be on pillows. During the day, try to raise the foot for 5 minutes in every 30 minutes. Walking helps the circulation, but standing in one place or sitting with the feet down for long periods is harmful.

Closed wounds (including abscesses and boils) which are infected:

Boils - and some abscesses - are red, raised painful lumps on the skin. They are most common on the groin, buttocks, armpits, back and upper legs. They may start as single lumps under the skin or in groups. They quickly become more painful as they increase in size. Once someone notices a red lump under the skin they should start using warm compresses over the area for 20 minutes four times a day. The warmth of the compresses will help the boil or abscess to "mature" or to form and harden and drain its contents. If they are having a great deal of pain and the boil or abscess continues to get bigger without draining (i.e. opening out onto the skin) they should seek help. The wound may require drainage and treatment with antibiotics.

Open wounds (including abscesses that are actively draining) which are infected:

If wounds are not cared for properly they can become infected. A wound is infected if:

- it becomes red, swollen, hot and painful
- it has pus either draining from it or visible under the skin
- it begins to smell bad.

The infection is spreading to other parts of the body if:

- it causes fever
- there is a red line above the wound
- the lymph nodes under the skin in the neck, armpits or groin become swollen and tender.

People should attend to open infected wounds with one of the following:

- a salt wash (one teaspoonful of salt in one cupful of clean water)
- hot compresses over the wound for 20 minutes, four times a day.

If there is pus or dead tissue, you should show the person how to clean it away:

- Use gentian violet solution on the wound before applying dressings.
- If the wound is on a hand or foot, soak it in a bucket of hot water with soap or potassium permanganate (one teaspoonful of potassium permaganate to a bucketful (4-5 litres) of clean or boiled water - do not exceed the recommended amount; if the solution is too concentrated it can burn or irritate the skin). Potassium permaganate compresses can also be applied to wounds elsewhere in the body. Be sure that any compress or water applied to the wound is not too hot, since damaged skin can easily burn.
- When it is not being soaked, keep the infected part at rest and elevated (raised above the level of the heart).
- If there is dead tissue, hydrogen peroxide can be used to rinse the wound.

Advice on washing or cleaning an infected wound and applying dressings

- Use gloves, plastic bags, or a big leaf when handling cleansing cloths or dressings to avoid touching blood from the wound, and wash your hands afterwards with soap and water.
- Wash around the edge of the wound first, then wash from the centre out to the edges using separate little pieces of clean cloth for each wipe if possible.
- Cover the area with a clean piece of cloth and bandage if the wound has pus or blood. If the wound is dry it can be left exposed to the air it will heal quicker this way.

Dressings are used to cover wounds to prevent them from becoming infected, to protect other people from infection, to keep medicines in place or to avoid painful contact with the environment.

- Never apply a dressing tightly.
- Make sure dressings are clean.

- Change the dressing at least once a day. Be sure to look for signs of infection.
- After changing the dressing, rinse the soiled cloth and bandages in water and soap and put them in the sun to dry or put them in boiling water for a short period and hang them to dry. If the dressings are not to be re-used, always dispose of them properly by burning them or putting them in a pit latrine.

If soil or dirt gets into the wound it can become infected with the bacteria that cause a serious disease called tetanus (lockjaw). You should therefore ensure that people are fully immunized against tetanus. Even if they have been immunized for tetanus before, they may still need further immunization. Advise people who are not immunized against tetanus to seek medical help immediately if they are wounded or develop open sores.

Infected scabies

Scabies is caused by a type of tick which cannot be easily seen. The disease spreads through direct physical contact with the infected person, through clothing and bedding. Scabies is one of the common illnesses which can be easily treated at home.

Scabies cause tiny bumps all over the body, but most commonly between the fingers, around the waist and on the penis and scrotum in males and around the vaginal opening in females. The bumps are very itchy. With scratching, they get infected and form sores with pus. In patients with AIDS, they get infected frequently. The infection causes fever and the lymph nodes under the armpit or groin become swollen and painful.

Scabies should be treated as early as possible. If one person in the family has scabies, the whole family should be treated, even if they do not have the symptoms. Advise the following:

- The whole body should be washed and scrubbed with soap and water and benzyl benzoate should be applied all over the body except the face, and left on the body overnight. Fresh clothes should be worn.
- Next morning, no bath should be taken and the medicine should again be applied all over the body. The same thing should be done in the evening.
- The second morning, a bath should be taken and fresh clothes should be worn.
- The used clothes and the towels should be boiled, washed and put in the sun. If the bedding cannot be washed, it should be put in the sun. These actions will kill the insect.

In addition, treat the infected sores as explained in treatment of wounds which are the other than washing or cleaning an infected wound.

Shingles

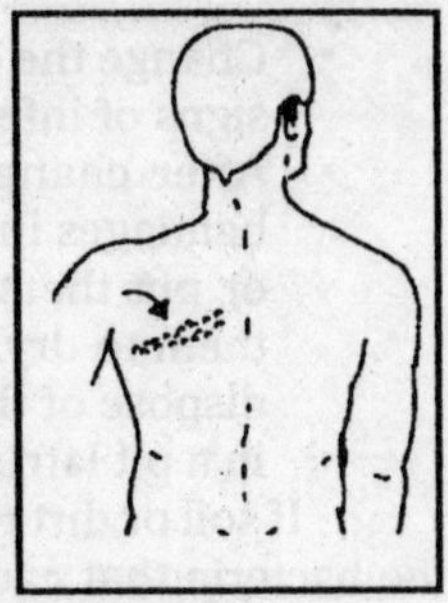

Shingles (herpes zoster) is a viral infection. Shingles is very common in people with AIDS and it may be one of the first symptoms they have of HIV infection or AIDS.

Shingles begins as a painful rash with small blisters, usually on the face, limbs or trunk. Shingles on the face may affect the eyes, causing pain and blurred vision. The blisters often combine, resulting in a large eroded or broken area, and there may be an intense burning feeling in the affected area. Healing takes place over several weeks and leaves discoloured areas on the skin.

The following measures may be helpful:

- Applying calamine lotion twice daily to relieve pain and itching promotes healing.
- Keeping the area dry and not letting clothes rub on them if possible.
- Wearing clean, loose-fitting, cotton clothing.
- Relieving pain with aspirine or paracetamol, but sometimes the pain may be so severe as to require stronger prescribed medicines, including pain killers and sedectives at night. For additional measures to control pain, see the section on pain in Chapter 8.
- Preventing infection by bathing the sores with warm salt water three or four times a day or applying gentian violet solution once a day, or antibiotic skin creams or ointments if available.
- Watching for signs of infection of the shingles sores such as redness or pus. If infection occurs, treat as indicated for infected wounds above.

The pain usually diminishes after three or four days. Unfortunately some people develop a persistent pain and scarring over the affected area. Rubbing creams on the scars or painful areas may help; medicines for pain such as aspirine or paracetamol may also be needed.

Allergic reactions

Allergic reactions to medicines are common in people with AIDS. These often appear suddenly and as skin rashes, redness, and itchy skin. If people think they may be having a reaction to a medicine they should immediately go to see the health care worker who prescribed it. Medicines that commonly cause reactions in people with AIDS include:

- anti-tuberculosis medicines

- antibiotics
- anti-cancer medicines.

See Chapter 8 for further details of possible reactions to anti-tuberculosis medicines.

Kaposi sarcoma

Kaposi sarcoma is a cancer of the cells in the blood vessels or lymph system. The cancer may begin as:

- discoloured (brown or purple) areas on the skin or in the mouth
- enlarged lymph glands which are not painful.

Both of these are a type of external cancer (affecting the outside of the body) and are mostly a problem for cosmetic reasons, but the cancer may go on to affect internal parts of the body causing the enlargement of internal organs or bleeding from the lungs or digestive tract. How Kaposi sarcoma will appear in a specific person and what its course will be are very difficult to predict. Some people have only mild complaints arising from the appearance of the lesions; others may become very ill as a result of the cancer.

Because of the variety of ways in which Kaposi sarcoma may appear and because of the numerous parts of the body that may be affected, this disease can be mistaken for many others. Once the diagnosis of Kaposi sarcoma is made, it indicates that the person has AIDS.

The specific care needed for the problems caused by Kaposi sarcoma will depend on where the cancer is situated and on what type of problems it is causing.

Bed sores

It is very important to prevent infections resulting from sores of any type that do not heal adequately. Included in this category are "bed sores". These are sores caused by breakdown of the skin due to pressure.

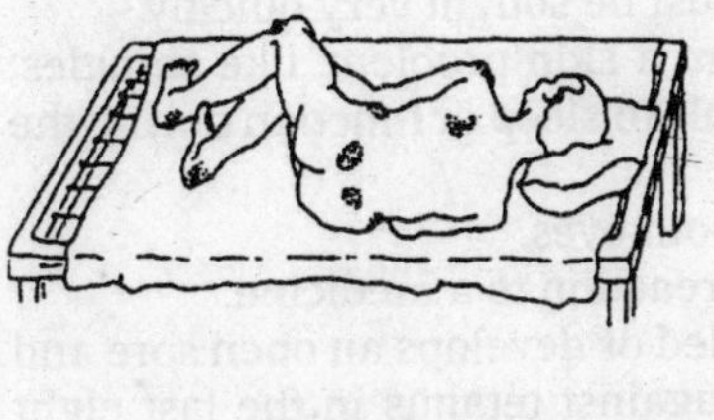

These chronic open sores appear in people who are so ill that they cannot roll over in bed, especially those who are very thin and weak. The sores form over bony parts of the body where the skin is pressed against the bedding. They most often occur on the buttocks, back, hips, elbows and feet.

To prevent bed sores in sick people you should advise them to:

- get out of bed as much as possible

- change position, when lying down, every two hours from one side onto the back, from the back onto the other side, and so on in order to prevent prolonged pressure and lack of circulation to any one area of the body; this is particularly important if an area of skin is already affected - the person may need help with turning in the home if they are very weak
- use soft bed sheets and padding, which should be hung to air daily and changed each time the bedding is soiled with urine, stools, vomit or sweat. Straighten the bedding often as lying on wrinkled bedding can hurt the skin

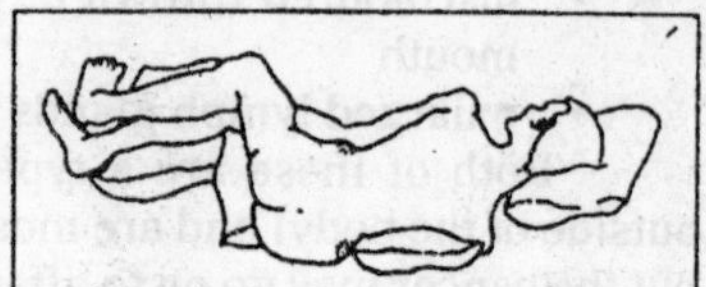

- put cushions under the body in such a way that the bony parts rub less (see illustration).
- eat as well as possible; extra vitamins may help.

A bedridden child who has a severe chronic illness should be held often on someones lap.

To treat bed sores, in addition to everything mentioned above, do the following:

- Wash all the sores with clean water mixed with a little salt or hydrogen peroxide. Gently remove any dead flesh. Protect them with sterile gauze bandages.

When sick people and their families must seek help

- If pus, redness or fever (indicating infection) accompanies the skin problem.
- If the wound has a bad smell, if brown or grey liquid oozes out, or if the skin around it turns black and forms air bubbles or blisters - this might be gangrene, a very dangerous condition. Medical help must be sought very quickly.
- If there is severe pain from a skin problem, like shingles, and the sick person is unable to sleep or function during the day.
- If shingles affects one or both eyes.
- If there is an allergic skin reaction to a medicine.
- If the sick person is wounded or develops an open sore and has not been immunized against tetanus in the last eight years.
- If the scabies does not respond to treatment.
- Kaposi sarcoma.
- Severe shingles.

NOTES ON SKIN PROBLEMS

MOUTH AND THROAT PROBLEMS

Problems and possible causes

Soreness in the mouth, usually accompanied by white patches on the tongue, is a common symptom in people with AIDS. Sometimes it progresses into the throat and oesophagus, causing painful swallowing, thereby interfering with eating and drinking. Other associated problems are blisters and sores on the lips, and dental problems. The following diseases may cause a sore mouth or throat in people with AIDS:

- thrush (yeast infection), resulting in white patches and surrounding redness, not only in the mouth but possibly in the throat and oesophagus
- oral herpes simplex (blisters and sores on the lips)
- malnutrition (cracks and sores on the mouth)
- Kaposi sarcoma of the mouth or throat
- dental problems
- hairy leukoplakia (also white patches in mouth).

What to do at home

Poor nutrition can cause problems in the mouth and can make existing problems worse. Encourage people to eat a healthy diet or take vitamin supplements. For additional information refer to the section on nutrition in this chapter and the section on medicines for nutrition problems in Chapter 8.

To help prevent problems in the mouth and throat, the mouth can be rinsed with warm salt water (half a teaspoonful of salt in a cupful of water), or with a mouthwash solution after eating and between meals. The wash should be swished gently in the mouth then spat out (not swallowed or it may upset the stomach and cause nausea).

General hints for dealing with a sore mouth:

- Eat soft foods rather than hard or crunchy foods.
- Eat bland not spicy foods.
- Use a straw for liquids and soups. This may help when taking in the food needed while preventing it from touching the sore areas.
- Cold foods, drinks or ice, if available, may help numb the mouth and relieve discomfort.
- Home remedies may help to make the ulcers less painful by forming a protective coating on the ulcer. The home remedies which may help are: - applying the bark of a banyan tree after grinding it into a smooth paste. - chewing some guava leaves before eating. These leaves have pectin in them, and this coats the ulcer making it less painful.

Thrush

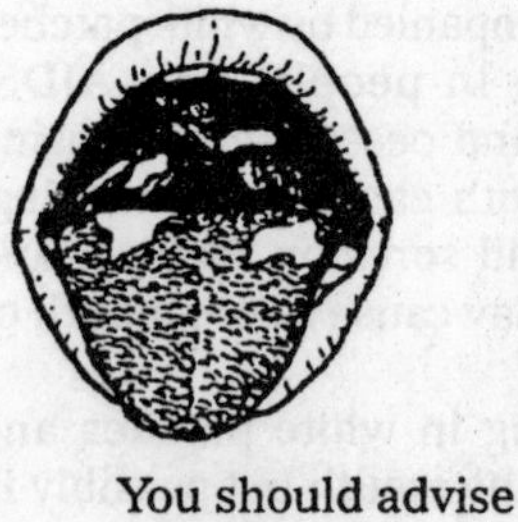

Thrush is a fungal infection that causes small white patches on the inside of the mouth and tongue. If the white plaques scrape off with a brush or a fingernail it is probably thrush. If it does not it may be another condition called hairy leukoplakia (described below).

You should advise someone with thrush to:

- gently scrub the tongue and gums with a soft toothbrush at least three or four times per day, then rinse the mouth with dilute mouthwash, or a salt water or lemon water rinse.
- suck a lemon if it is not too painful - the acid of the lemon slows down the growth of the fungus.

- apply gentian violet solution three or four times a day-gentian violet solution is prepared by dissolving 1 teaspoonful of gentian violet crystals in half a litre of clean water.
- chew garlic or eat yogurt.

If necessary, you may prescribe antifungal oral suspensions or lozenges given three or four times a day. In some people, thrush affects not only the mouth but the entire oesophagus causing pain on swallowing and a burning sensation in the chest. See the section on medicines for fungal infections in Chapter 8 for information on the use of these medicines.

Hairy leukoplakia

Hairy leukoplakia may look like thrush. However, it does not cause pain, it will not scrub off the tongue or gums, and it commonly makes vertical ridges on the edges of the tongue. It is mentioned here only so that you know that it can be confused with thrush. There is no need for a specific treatment for this condition. It will not interfere with the ability to eat or with a persons general comfort. The main point is to not use too many medicines for thrush if in fact the problem is hairy leukoplakia.

Herpes simplex sores

These are painful blisters on the lips, which may appear after a fever. In people with AIDS these sores may appear even without a fever and may last a long time. Gentian violet solution (made as described in the previous section on thrush) can be applied to the herpes sores on the lips and mouth. Although the strong purple colour may bother some people, the solution can help in preventing the sores from becoming infected.

Dental problems

Thorough cleaning of the teeth and gums is important, preferably after each meal. Many people with AIDS suffer from inflammation of the gums, tooth abscesses and infection. For this reason, people should be encouraged to make regular visits to a dentist when possible, and to be particularly careful about oral hygiene, being sure to brush the teeth and clean between the teeth (using dental floss or toothpicks) to remove food particles.

If someone does not have a toothbrush, they can use a tooth-cleaning stick.

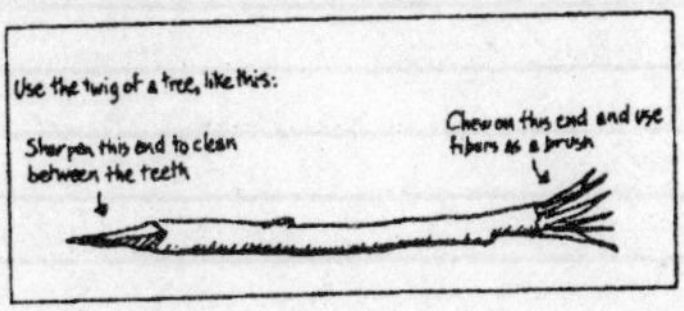

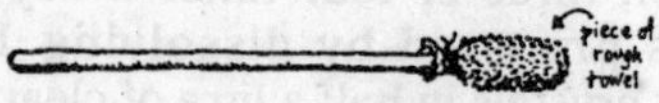

Or, they can tie a piece of towel around the end self stick and use it as a toothbrush.

If toothpaste is not available, a tooth-cleaning powder can be made by mixing salt and bicarbonate of soda (or ashes) in equal amounts. To make it stick, the brush should be wetted before being put in the powder. This mixture works just as well as commercially available toothpaste for cleaning teeth.

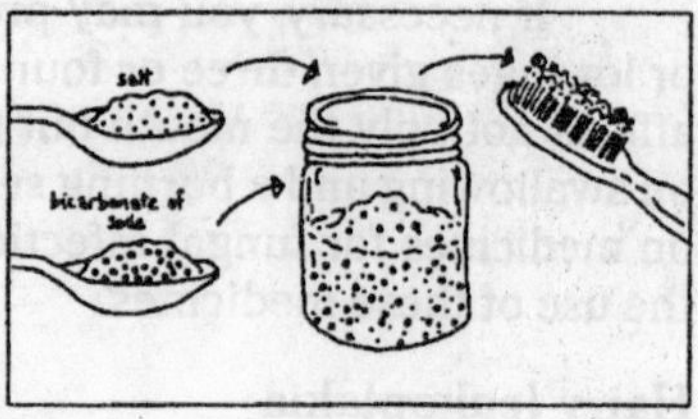

In case of toothaches, a pain reliever like aspirin or paracetamol can be taken. See Chapter 8 for specific information about these medicines. Chewing cloves may also help.

Protective foods rich in vitamin, especially eggs, meat, beans, dark green vegetables, and fruits like oranges, lemons, and tomatoes should be eaten. Sweet, sticky and stringy foods that get stuck between the teeth should be avoided.

When sick people and their families must seek help

- If the sick person is unable to drink or is unable to swallow properly.
- If there are symptoms of oesophageal thrush such as a burning pain in the chest or a deep pain on swallowing.
- If tooth infection is severe with fever~ swelling;, pus, etc.

NOTES ON SORE MOUTH AND THROAT

COUGHING AND DIFFICULTY IN BREATHING

Problems and possible causes

Respiratory problems, particularly lung infections, are common in people with AIDS and can be quite serious. The most common symptoms are chronic cough, shortnes of breath, chest pain, and increased production of mucus (also called sputum).

The most common causes in AIDS of respiratory problems include:

- colds and flu
- bronchitis
- pneumonia
- tuberculosis (see Chapter 7)
- heart problems.

What to do at home

People should be made aware of the signs and symptoms that are of concern including:

- the onset of a fever or a change in the regular fever pattern of the sick person
- blood in the sputum
- a sudden or rapid worsening in their ability to breathe or catch their breath after normal activity
- a change in the colour of their sputum from clear to grey, yellow or green
- pain in the chest.

The following advice may help to decrease respiratory problems.

- Keeping active by walking about, turning in bed and sitting up. This encourages the lungs to drain.
- Other measures which encourage drainage of the lungs include massage or gentle patting on the back of the chest over the lungs. Someone in the home can do this, especially for younger children.
- If pain is felt in the chest or ribs during coughing, a pillow or hand should be held tightly over the area that hurts when coughing. This helps make the cough less painful.

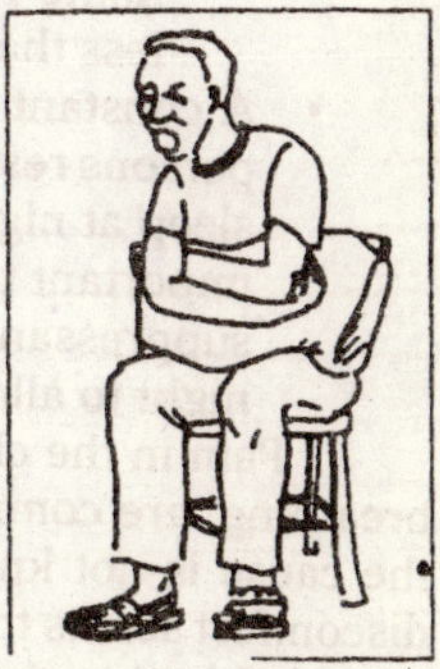

- During the day it may be beneficial to cough and clear the lungs at least four times a day. Even though coughing may cause discomfort, it is an important way to clean the lungs of the accumulated mucus and disease-causing bacteria.

Thus, anyone with lung problems should be encouraged to cough.

The following points should be remembered:

- The bacteria or infectious agents in the sick persons sputum can be passed on to other people through the air, especially when coughing. When anyone is coughing, they should always cover their mouth with their hand or with a cloth which can be cleaned or disposed of.
- All homes and other places where people meet should be ventilated -make sure there is a way in and a way out for fresh air.
- For loosening the mucus and ease any kind of cough, people with cough should be advised to:
  - drink lots of water. This works better than any kind of medicine.
  - breathe hot water vapors.
  - Sit down on a chair with a bucket of hot water at your feet. Place a sheet over your head and cover the bucket so that you can inhale the vapors as they rise. Breathe the vapors deeply for 15 minutes. Repeat this several times in a day.
- An irritating cough can sometimes be relieved with safe cough remedies, for example:
  - Soothe the throat by sipping warm tea with sugar or honey.
  - Use a safe, home-made remedy to soothe the throat and relieve the cough.
  - Commercial remedies may also be useful although they are often expensive and usually work no better than home remedies. These should be avoided in children less than five years of age.
- A constant cough can be very tiring and interfere with a persons rest. If coughing keeps someone from being able to sleep at night a cough suppressant can be prescribed. It is important to cough, so do not encourage the use of cough suppressant during the day. They should only be used at night to allow someone to rest.

Pain in the chest without signs of infection, and difficulty in breathing, are common problems in people with AIDS. Very often the cause is not known. Warm compresses to the area where the discomfort seems to be centred may be helpful. Additional hints are provided in this chapter under the section on pain. Medicines like aspirin or paracetamol may be useful at times. Paracetamol is safer for children. The dosages are described in the section on medicines for pain in Chapter 8. It is important that the things done to help relieve the pain will also help someone in their efforts to keep active, moving and coughing.

When someone is experiencing difficulty in breathing the following advice might help:

- Lie with pillows under the head, or with the head of the bed raised on blocks.
- Sit leaning forward with the elbows on the knees or on a low table.
- Have someone else there to comfort and help. Difficulty in breathing can be very frightening.

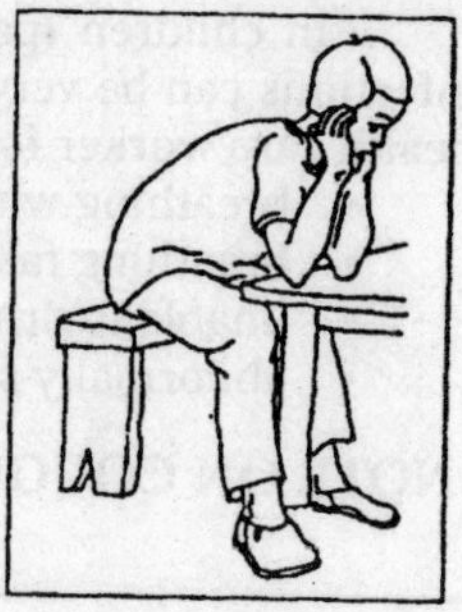

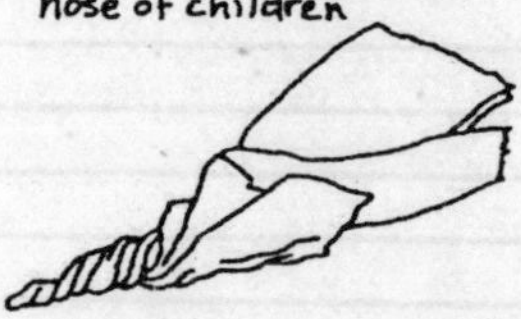

In children with respiratory problems it is important to clear the nose if it is blocked, and especially if the congestion interferes with the ability to eat or to be breast-fed.

Dry or thick sticky mucus can be softened and removed with a wick made of clean material or tissue, moistened in salt water (a quarter of a teaspoonful in a cup of water).

If a lung infection with cough is present, it is important that plenty of fluids are drunk: first, to replace the extra fluids lost through the lungs by rapid breathing and, second, to help keep the mucus in the lungs from becoming too dry and sticky and more difficult to cough out. Remind parents that fast or difficult breathing in children may be dangerous and needs medical treatment quickly.

Encourage children with respiratory problems to take more fluids by increasing the frequency of breast-feeding or by giving additional fluids by spoon or cup.

If the problems experienced with coughing, chest pain, or other respiratory symptoms are chronic (lasting more than three weeks) and do not respond to antibiotic treatment, tuberculosis may be the cause and should always be considered (see Chapter 7).

When sick people and their families must seek help

You should advise people to seek help if the sick person has a cough or difficulty in breathing and:

- sudden high fever develops
- they are in severe pain or discomfort
- the colour of the sputum changes to grey, yellow or green
- the sputum has blood in it

- they have had a cough for more than three weeks, especially if it also involves spitting up blood, pain in the chest or difficulty in breathing
- severe difficulty in breathing.

In children (particularly below the age of five) respiratory infections can be very serious. All children should be brought to a health care worker for immediate attention if they are:

- breathing with difficulty or with noises from the chest
- breathing faster than usual
- unable to drink because of problems with breathing
- abnormally sleepy or difficult to wake.

NOTE ON COUGHING AND DIFFICULTY BREATHING

GENITAL PROBLEMS

Other sexually transmitted diseases (STDs) and opportunistic infections of the genital area are common in both men and women with AIDS, and may recur on numerous occasions. STDs that cause ulcerative lesions promote the transmission of HIV through sex. Effective diagnosis, care and education about genital problems are, therefore, crucial to both the prevention of HIV transmission and to the care of people with HIV infection.

In women, the genital area includes the external and internal labia of the vagina, the surrounding skin surface, the opening of the vagina (which is called the vulva) and the vagina itself.

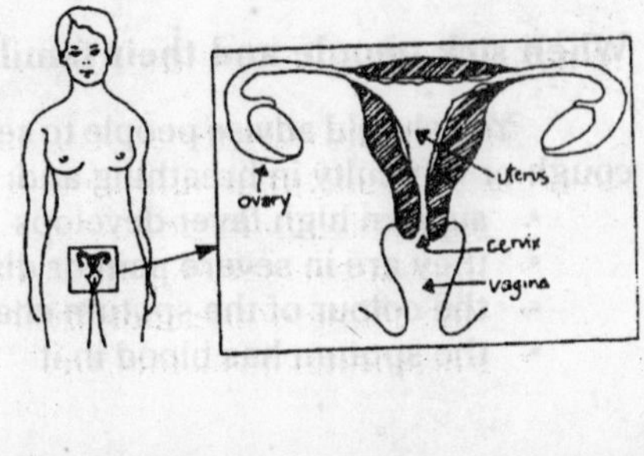

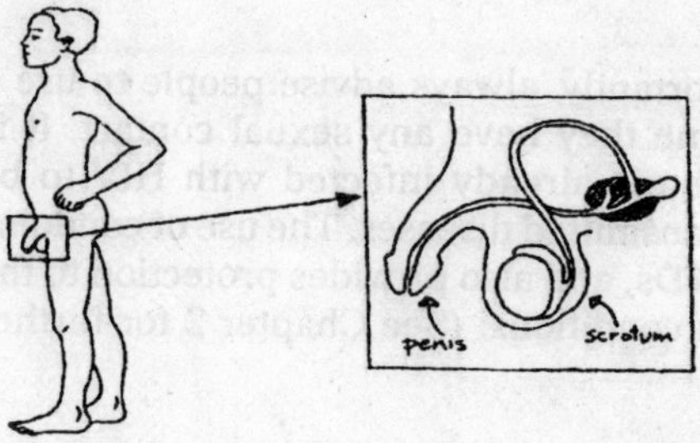

The genital area in the male consists of the penis, which may be circumcised or not, the scrotum containing the testicles and the surrounding skin. If uncircumcised, the end of the penis will be covered with loose skin which can be pulled back. This is called the foreskin.

The rectal area and the inguinal areas of the groin in men and women may also be involved in genital problems such as infections, rashes, warts or sores.

Problems and possible causes

Infections of the genital area, including certain STDs, are common in both men and women with AIDS. They often cause pain and discomfort.

There are six common ways that such genital problems appear in men and women:

- an unusual discharge (a mucus or pus-like substance) from the vagina
- an unusual discharge from the urethral opening of the penis
- open sores or ulcers in the genital, groin or rectal areas, which sometimes start as blisters
- a rash in or around the genital area
- warts in the genital area or around the anus
- swollen glands in the groin.

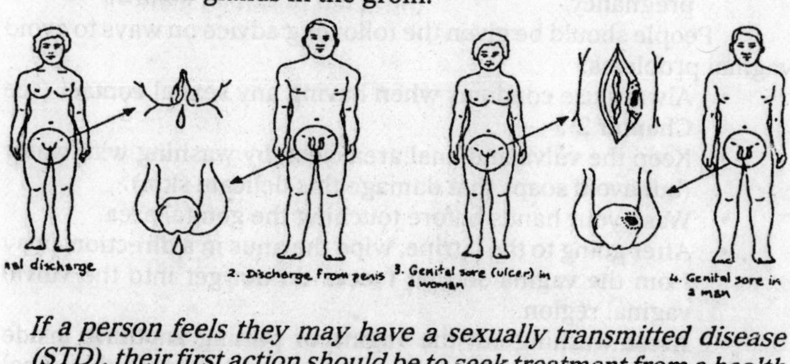

If a person feels they may have a sexually transmitted disease (STD), their first action should be to seek treatment from a health care worker where avail- able, before attempting any form of home treatment. Do not have sexual relations until treatment has been completed.

What to do at home

Firstly and very importantly, always advise people to use a condom each and every time they have any sexual contact. It is dangerous for someone who is already infected with HIV to be exposed to other sexually transmitted diseases. The use of condoms offers protection from all STDs, and also provides protection to the partners of those with such conditions. (See Chapter 2 for further information on safer sex.)

Vaginal discharge

All women normally have a small amount of vaginal discharge which is clear, milky-white or slightly yellow and varies in amount and appearance over the course of the monthly menstrual cycle. Any change in this normal discharge, particularly if it is accompanied by either an unpleasant smell, itching, a burning sensation during urination, pain in the lower abdomen, soreness and sometimes fever, is probably caused by a sexually transmitted infection such as gonorrhoca, chlamydia or trichomonas..

Vaginal infections are important because:

- They may be passed on to others during sexual intercourse.
- Sexually transmitted infections (e.g. gonorrhoca, chlamydia) are particularly likely to spread from the genital area to the upper reproductive tract causing pelvic inflammatory disease. This may even lead to abscesses with severe cramps and pains in the abdomen, with the result that such infections become difficult to treat, even with strong medicine, and can be life-threatening.
- They increase the risk of acquiring, or passing on, HIV infection during sex.
- They may be transmitted to an unborn child during pregnancy.

People should be given the following advice on ways to avoid vaginal problems:

- Always use condoms when having any sexual contact (see Chapter 2).
- Keep the vulva and anal area clean by washing with water (but avoid soaps that damage this delicate skin).
- Wash your hands before touching the genital area.
- After going to the latrine, wipe the anus in a direction away from the vagina so that faeces do not get into the vulva/ vaginal region.
- Avoid washing out the vagina or putting anything inside unless advised by a health care worker. Anyone with vaginal discharge should be examined by a health care worker.

Urethral discharge in men

Pus or mucus discharge from the opening of the urethra, often accompanied by burning when passing urine, is usually a sign of an STD. Anyone with these symptoms should be examined by a health care worker.

Genital sores

Open sores or lesions on the genitals may be caused by an STD. As with any open wound (see the section on skin problems in this chapter) an additional infection may occur. People with open sores should be advised to:

- see a health worker
- always use condoms when having any sexual contact (see Chapter 2) and be shown how to use condoms properly
- keep the affected area clean with soap and water
- between washings keep the wound dry
- watch for signs of infection, and seek help if redness, pus or swelling are seen, or if the sores become painful.

Genital warts

Genital warts are very common, are infectious, and can be caught by sexual contact, then passed on to other people in the same way. They are often larger, spread more quickly and are more difficult to treat in people with AIDS. In women, they appear as skin-coloured lumps or swellings on the outside and inside of the vagina, and the area around the anus, while in men they appear particularly under the foreskin and around the anus. If they get rubbed by clothing or damaged they may become sore (inflamed), infected and may even bleed.

Encourage people to seek early treatment from a health care worker for this condition. Local treatment of the warts provided by a health care worker can be effective if it is applied before the warts are too big. If a person waits too long and the warts become quite big it may be necessary to have them cut out, a surgical procedure which has risks associated with it. Warts that are damaged may become infected. If infection occurs they should be treated like any open wound in the genital area.

Herpes

Herpes is a viral infection that many people get around their mouths or genital area. It tends to remain latent (hidden away), under the control of the bodys defences. It occasionally appears as blisters which break down to give painful ulcers which heal slowly by themselves. In people with AIDS, the blisters appear more frequently, spread over a wider area and sometimes do not heal at all. They can be very difficult to treat.

If herpes is diagnosed, advise the person to bathe the affected area with salt solution consisting of a teaspoonful of ordinary cooking salt in half a litre of clean water. They should do this often, every two or three hours if possible. Between times the affected area should be kept dry. Calamine, talcum or starch powder may also be applied to the sore.

Candidiasis

Candidal infections are common but they are particularly frequent and more difficult to cure in people with AIDS. In women, they produce a curdy vaginal discharge and cause redness and soreness of the vulva that is accompanied by severe itching. The skin around the vulva may break down and bleed, particularly if scratched. Candidiasis also occurs often and severely in men with AIDS. The foreskin and the area underneath it become very sore and red. There may be a yellow discharge under the foreskin. The skin of the penis, scrotum, and around the anus sometimes becomes red, sore and itchy.

Candidiasis is not sexually transmitted but is often brought on by the use of antibiotics for the treatment of other conditions, or simply because the person with AIDS has lowered resistance to the fungi that cause it. The organisms are always present in the genital area but are not normally a problem because the bodys defences keep them from growing out of control.

If someone is experiencing candidiasis repeatedly, the following approach may help to alleviate discomfort, to prevent the onset of a new infection (which will occur, for example, as a result of taking antibiotics given for another problem) and possibly to decrease the intensity of an existing infection:

- Apply gentian violet to the vulva and vaginal area or the affected male genital area. To prepare a gentian violet solution dissolve one or two teaspoonfuls of gentian violet crystals in one litre of clean water. Apply once daily for three days. Gentian violet solution should be applied internally or externally to the affected area using a soaked piece of clean cotton wool, cloth or gauze. This should be done for at least three days or until the symptoms improve - if this does not happen then the person must see a health care worker. People should be advised that gentian violet stains clothing and sheets a purple colour.

A rash on the penis or under the foreskin will often respond to soaking in .1 dilute salt and water solution. Dissolve a teaspoonful of salt in a glass or jam jar of water. Pull back the foreskin, put the penis in the water and soak for 5 minutes. Repeat 2 or 3 times a day.

If this does not work, carry out the same procedure using gentian violet solution (1/2 teaspoonful gentian violet in 1 litre of clean water). If the rash does not clear up in 3-4 days the person should ask advice from a health care worker.

A person who experiences candidiasis repeatedly should learn to recognize the signs of an infection and begin the treatment at home while it is still in the early stages.

Menstrual problems

Loss of menstruation and irregular or erratic bleeding occur in many illnesses including AIDS If a woman loses a lot of weight her periods may stop altogether or become infrequent. Loss of menstrual bleeding can have many causes (including pregnancy) and is often seen in women with AIDS. This should be assessed in order to plan for the future care of the woman (see Chapter 5). If a woman misses one or two periods, she should be encouraged to go to the health centre to be examined. If pregnancy is not the cause then the reason for the loss of menstruation should, where possible, be determined.

Always remember that a woman may feel that loss of menstruation represents a loss of capacity to bear children or a loss of femininity and may feel sad or even depressed. You can help such a person to fight this loss of self-esteem by reassuring her that loss of menstruation is experienced by many women for a wide variety of reasons. Women should be encouraged to be with friends, to involve themselves in the people and activities around them, and to remember that they are still worthwhile and have a great deal to give.

When sick people and their families must seek help

- If an STD is suspected.
- If difficulty or pain in passing urine is experienced.
- If genital warts are present.
- If genital ulcers are present.
- If there is an unusual vaginal discharge that is foul-smelling, itchy, very plentiful, or green, yellow or grey in colour.
- If a pain develops in a woman's lower abdomen, particularly if it is accompanied by a fever.
- If a woman's periods stop or become irregular or erratic.
- If there is a discharge from the penis.
- If there is swelling and/or pain in the scrotum.

NOTES ON GENITAL PROBLEM

NUTRITION PROBLEMS

Problems and possible causes

AIDS almost always cases severe weight loss, even in people who eat good food. There are many reasons for this, including:

- not enough nutritious foods available
- painful or difficult swallowing because of:
  - oral or oesophageal thrush
  - mouth sores such as the blisters caused by herpes simptems
  - Kaposi sarcoma lesions in the mouth (purple lesions which can occur on gums or palate)
  - inflammation of the gums or infections of the gums and teeth (redness, pus or swelling of the gums); these can be caused by a lack of vitamin C (found primarily in citrus fruits and in dark green leafy vegetables).
- nausea and vomiting
- chronic diarrhoea
- tuberculosis (see Chapter 8)
- depression or anxiety
- fever from any cause.

What to do at home

A sick person has an even greater need for food than a healthy person. People should be encouraged to think about the foods that will help make them healthy, rather than worry about foods that are not considered to be good for them.

The same foods that are good for you when you are healthy and good for you when you are sick.

All of the foods you are familiar with will fall into one of the following three groups. Everyone should try to eat food from each of these groups at every meal.

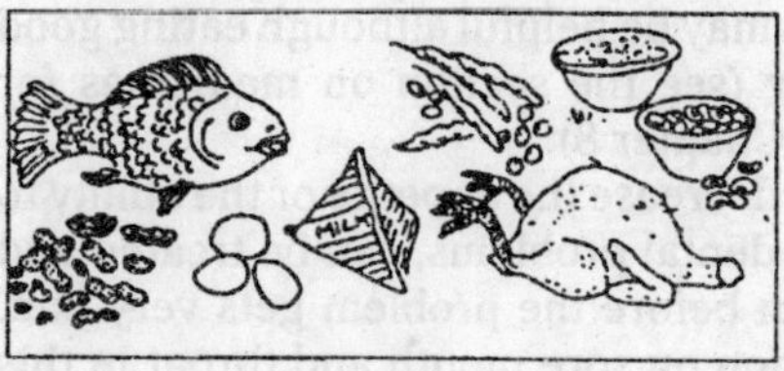

1. Body-building foods: These include peas, beans, soya, groundnuts, nuts, eggs, meat, fish, cheese and milk. These foods are rich in protein and contain iron and calcium.

2. Energy-giving foods: These include potatoes, yams, plantains, sugar, wheat, rice, millet, maize, animal fats and vegetable oils.

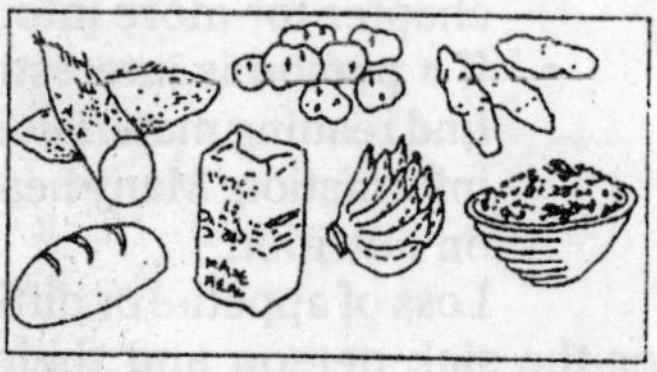

3. Foods that protect the body from infection (vitamin-rich foods): These include all fruits and vegetables, especially dark green leafy vegetables and orang coloured vegetables and fruits. Cooking for too long destroys vitamins so these foods should be cooked or steamed lightly, and the cooking water used as a soup or sauce.

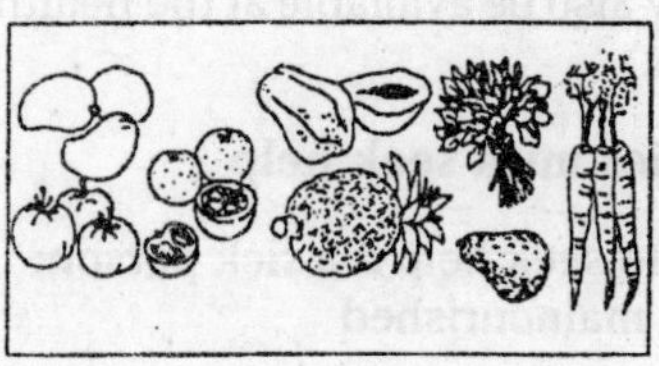

As mentioned in the section on diarrhoea in this chapter, correct preparation and storage of foods should ensure that they are clean and safe and do not cause disease. This is especially important for infants.

General hints for people who are having trouble eating or maintaining their weight and strength

- Eat small amounts often. Foods that can be eaten with the

fingers are easier to manage, particularly if the person is weak.

- To supplement a regular diet of nutritious foods, vegetable oil or groundnut paste can be added to food.
- Raw vegetables are not very digestible and can easily be contaminated, so they are not advisable.
- If someone is experiencing nausea or vomiting, preparing the foods in liquid or semi-liquid form may help.
- If persistent diarrhoea is present, use soft or mashed foods and avoid irritating foods, for example pepper and raw vegetables.
- Drink plenty of fluids and watch for dehydration (see the section on diarrhoea in this chapter).
- Taking vitamin tablets may be helpful although eating good foods is always better (see the section on medicines for nutrition problems in Chapter 8).
- Certain problems that decrease the appetite or the ability to eat, such as thrush or dental problems, can be treated and action should be taken before the problem gets very bad. Refer back to the section on sore mouth and throat in this chapter for more information about this.
- If a person is interested or has more questions, help them find reading materials in their own language that give further information. Many health centres have books and pamphlets on nutrition.

Loss of appetite or difficulty in eating can be very distressing for the sick person and their family and might make them feel helpless and ineffective. It may help if they can discuss this with a health care worker. A nutritionist may also be available at the health centre to provide further information.

When sick people and their families must seek help

People should be encouraged to seek help if a sick person:

- becomes dehydrated or very malnourished
- is suddenly unable to eat
- starts to have severe abdominal pain with or without vomiting
- severe vomiting.

NOTES ON NUTRITIONAL PROBLEMS

NAUSEA AND VOMITING

Problems and possible causes

Nausea and vomiting can be important problems for people with AIDS. These symptoms may be caused by:

- medicines
- infections
- a problem with the stomach or intestines
- Kaposi sarcoma in the intestines
- HIV infection itself.

In some people with AIDS, nausea and vomiting are very short-lived, and go away by themselves or after treatment of the cause. In others, they are chronic or long-lasting and become a part of daily life.

What to do at home

If a person is having trouble with nausea and vomiting advise them to:

- avoid cooking smells if possible
- watch out for dehydration (see the section on diarrhoea in this chapter)
- talk to a health care worker, who may prescribe medicine to

control the symptoms if they are very severe, in order to allow the person to eat. See the section on medicines for nausea and vomiting in Chapter 8 for further details.

If someone is vomiting severely they should:

- not eat any food or drink any fluids for one or two hours
- then gradually start drinking room-temperature water, oral rehydration solution, weak tea, or other clear liquids (about two tablespoonfuls an hour for two to three hours), or suck ice in small amounts
- then increase the amount of fluids to four to six tablespoonfuls an hour for two to three hours; the amount can be increased as desired but people should force themselves to keep taking fluids to make up for what they have lost.

As the nausea decreases, people should increase the amount and types of foods they eat. It may be best to start with small quantities of dry, plain foods such as bread, rice or cassava.

Frequent care of the mouth will remove the foul taste caused by vomiting anal freshen it. This can include rinsing the mouth with water, or gently cleaning the tongue and gums with a soft toothbrush or cloth at least three or four times a day, then rinsing with dilute mouthwash or lemon water rinse.

Ventilating or freshening a room may make a person feel better and less nauseated.

It is also a good idea for people to identify and reduce the things that seem to make them feel nauseated, such as specific odours, medicines, or foods (high-fat foods, for example).

A cool compress applied to the forehead, or other things which help someone to relax, may be useful.

Vomit can be cleaned without fear of HIV, as the virus is not present in vomitus.

When sick people and their families must seek help

- If vomiting occurs repeatedly and fluids cannot be kept down - in such cases the sick person is at risk of becoming severely dehydrated
- If regular vomiting lasts more than 24 hours, particularly if it is accompanied by pain in the abdomen.
- If the person has a fever in addition to the vomiting.
- If the sick person is vomiting violently, especially if the vomit is dark green, brown, or smells like faeces.
- If the vomit contains blood.

NOTES ON NAUSEA AND VOMITING

ANXIETY AND DEPRESSION

Problems and possible causes

The diagnosis of HIV infection or AIDS is usually a crisis for the infected person their family and their friends. When people receive the news of HIV or AIDS the begin to experience the psychological reactions described in Chapter 3, starting with shock. They may feel confused and that their mind is in constant turmoil. How someone reacts and behaves after this initial shock depends on many things, for example how they have dealt with stresses in their life before and what types of support they can get for emotional and social problems. Resources that are available within a culture should be used to deal with anxiety and depression.

Anxiety (a feeling of nervousness, fear and dead) and depression (a feeling of sadness and hopelessness) are normal if someone has been told that they have HIV infection or AIDS, and is trying to cope with it. It is when these feelings are very intense or last a long time, so that normal daily activities are interrupted, that they are considered abnormal.

The physical symptoms experienced with either anxiety or depression can be dramatic and may lead people to think that they are physically ill. Learning to recognize their own symptoms allows people to distinguish between those which are caused by anxiety or depression and those that may indicate the onset of a infection or illness.

Possible explanations for symptoms which resemble those of either anxiety or depression include:

- Infections
- side-effects of some medicines
- malnutrition.

Anxiety

Anxiety, the feeling of nervousness, can have both physical and menta' symptoms.

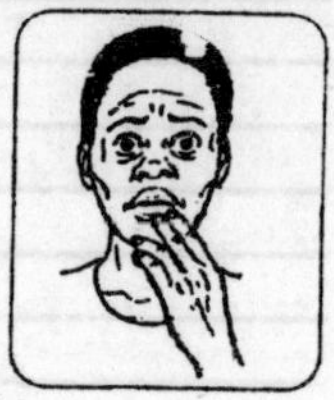

The symptoms include:

- lack of appetite
- feeling short of breath
- shaking
- a sensation that the heart is pounding
- sweating
- tingling sensations, for example in the hands
- feeling faint
- difficulty in sleeping
- a feeling of being out of control
- difficulty in concentrating
- feeling very worried
- feeling irritable or nervous.

Other symptoms include headache, which is discussed in the section on pain.

Depression

When someone has HIV infection or AIDS they experience many losses in a very short period of time. Examples of this might include loss of health, loss of physical beauty, loss of job or ability to function in the community, loss of mobility, loss of eyesight. For all these losses a person will grieve and will at times feel very unhappy.

A person may experience depression in the following ways:

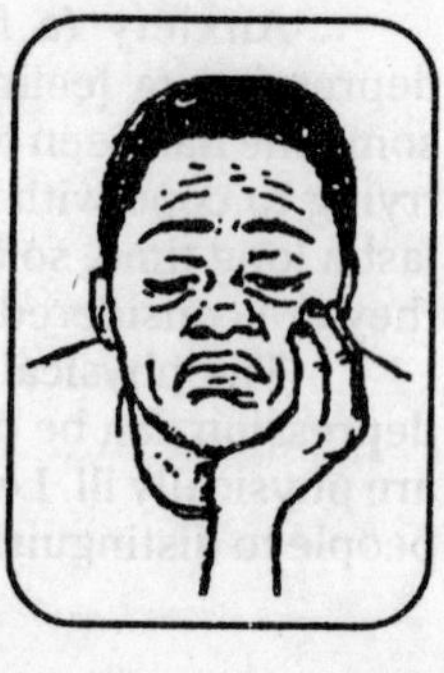

- a feeling of hopelessness
- feeling tired and generally without energy
- inability to find pleasure and the sense that everything is a chore
- irritability
- inability to concentrate and poor memory
- waking up early in the morning or having trouble getting to sleep at night

- eating too much or being unable to eat
- wanting to be alone
- not talking.

Most people get depressed from time to time. Certainly if someone is facing AIDS it is likely they will be depressed for hours or even days at a time. Periods depression may come and go, alternating with periods when the person doesn't el depressed at all.

Depression can be more than a passing mood and is something to be concerned out if it occurs very frequently or is very intense. This sort of depression can make difficult to deal with everyday life, and ultimately can lead people to harm themselves or to consider suicide, especially those who are isolated and those who have suffered considerable losses and stress.

What to do at home

Treatment of anxiety and depression varies from culture to culture. In many communities, support for such problems is often provided by trusted elders in the family and through traditional systems. Together with the suggestions made below, as a health care worker you should help people with AIDS to find the best support in the community to help them overcome anxiety and depression.

Chapters 3, 4 and 5 provide information on emotional support including psychological support and care of the dying. This information will also help to provide care for anxiety and depression.

The process discussed in the section on psychological reactions to AIDS in chapter 3 is very important here. You can give people an opportunity to progress through the stages of grief simply by encouraging them to talk, and than by listening to them. It is not expected that you will have answers; it is enough that you are there. Encourage them to express their thoughts and feelings.

If you are aware of others in the community with AIDS or with any other chronic or terminal illness who have adjusted to their life and are willing to speak about it, consider finding ways for them to be in contact with those who are anxious or depressed. This contact with others with similar problems (peer contact) can great support and inspiration.

The support you can give people with AIDS will also depend on the resources that the family and the community have to address major concerns such as child care, finances and transport. Become familiar with any support groups in you community or region which can provide help to people with AIDS and those who care for them. If no such groups are available, start one!

Help sick people plan activities on a daily or weekly basis. This can help them to fight the sense that their life is out of control or that they cannot accomplish anything. The important point here is that these plans should be realistic in terms of the persons abilities and time.

Encourage sick people and their family members to learn how to relax. This is a skill that takes time to master, but it can be very helpful. It is good to have both physical and mental relaxing activities.

Although alcohol and other "drugs" may seem to help people relax, if used in excess they may actually result in a worsening of the anxiety and depression over time.

The use of medicines for treating the symptoms of anxiety can be very helpful and may make an enormous difference to someone's ability to function. However such medicines can have serious side-effects so their use should be carefully supervised.

When sick people and their families must seek help

If the family or the patient believe that the anxiety or depression is severe enough that the patient may commit suicide, otherwise harm themselves, or harm someone else.

If there is a prolonged disruption in the sick person's ability to function, such as in sleeping, eating, relating to their family or friends, or going about their daily life, that is not explained by any physical disability they may have.

NOTES ON ANXIETY AND DEPRESSION

PAIN

Problems and possible causes

For some people in the later stages of AIDS, physical pain becomes a part of daily life. For others it is only occasional and easily controlled.

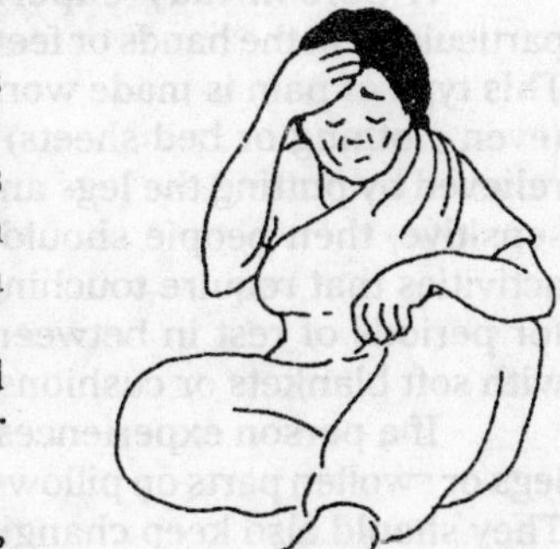

The causes of pain are many and include:

- immobility
- infections, such as herpes zoster
- swelling of the extremities (caused by poor circulation brought on by Kaposi sarcoma or problems with the heart)
- headache alone or associated with meningitis or encephalitis
- nerve problems including pain with or without weakness
- Psychological or emotional causes such as depression and anxiety which may increase the sense of being in physical pain
- side-effects of medicines.

What to do at home

In attempting to control and relieve pain, people will need to know that pain is also influenced by the person's emotional state and can be frightening. The sick person may need extra reassurance and care.

Encourage people to look out for any clues as to what increases or relieves pain.

People can take an active role in controlling their pain. For example by:

- learning deep and regular breathing techniques, which may help them to relax
- learning to deal with pain through distraction and lessening of their anxiety see the section on anxiety and depression in this chapter
- taking medicines for pain according to an organized schedule - this can help people to feel more in control and reassure them that the pain will not become too great before medicine is taken

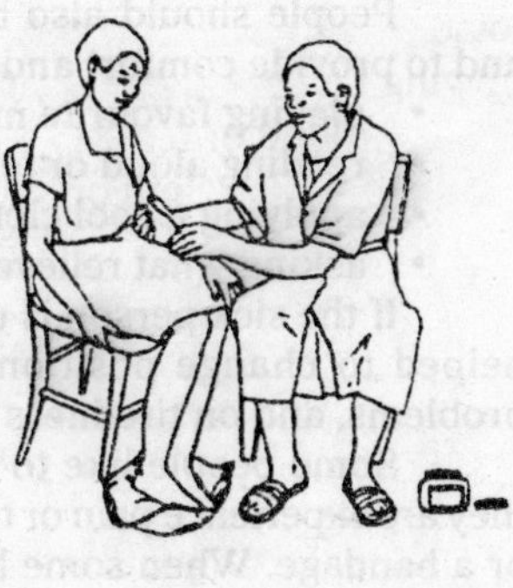

- engaging in physical activity or receiving gentle massage - both of these can be helpful for some types of pain
- imagining or remembering a favourite place or event.

A person may experience a strong burning sensation, particularly in the hands or feet, which may be due to nerve problems. This type of pain is made worse by extremes of temperature, touch (even clothing or bed sheets) and dryness. The pain is sometimes relieved by putting the legs and feet in water. If the skin seems to be sensitive, then people should plan things so that all the care and activities that require touching are done at the same time, to allow for periods of rest in between. The sick persons bed can be lined with soft blankets or cushions.

If a person experiences any swelling, they should raise their legs or swollen parts on pillows, or raise the foot of the bed on blocks. They should also keep changing their body position.

Treatment for pain of all types may include mild medicines for pain (analgesics) which are commonly used in the home, such as:

- aspirin
- paracetamol.

There are other stronger medicines which people can take for pain but these should only be taken with the advice of a health care worker. See the section on medicines for pain in Chapter 8 for further details.

It is important that the sick person takes the mild pain medicines regularly, at least every eight hours, if the problem is long-lasting or chronic. Waiting until the pain is very severe before taking the medicine makes it less likely to work effectively.

If someone is caring for a person with AIDS who is in pain, you should give them advice which will help them to keep the environment as calm as possible. For example, you could advise them to:

- talk slowly to the sick person, and use gentle tones
- approach the person slowly and quietly
- avoid using bright lights
- ask others to be quiet and gentle in the presence of the sick person.

People should also be encouraged to talk with the person, and to provide comfort and distraction from the pain, perhaps by:

- playing favourite music quietly
- reading aloud or telling stories
- applying a cool cloth on the forehead, or giving massage
- asking what relieves the pain and then doing it.

If the sick person is unable to move unaided, they should be helped to change position frequently (see the sections on skin problems, and on tiredness and weakness in this chapter).

Some people like to be wrapped in a blanket or cloth when they are experience pain or to have the painful area wrapped in cloths or a bandage. When some lifts a child who is in pain, the palms of the hands should be used rather than the fingertips (which can sometimes feel like a pinch).

When sick people and their families must seek help

If the pain becomes unbearable or is associated with new symptoms such as a severe headache or weakness.

If there is a sudden or recent occurrence of pain in the hands or feet. People need to be certain it is not due to another illness or medicines for other disease (see Chapter 8, section on tuberculosis).

If there is a persistent headache lasting over two weeks, a severe headache whiz is getting rapidly worse and is not relieved by the usual ways of dealing with pain, a headache associated with vomiting or a headache that affects the sick person ability to think or move.

NOTES ON PAIN

TIREDNESS AND WEAKNESS

Problems and possible causes

AIDS can often make a person feel very tired and weak, particularly in the later stages of the illness. This can have many causes and to some extent is unavoidable. It is important to advise people to do what they can to keep their strength up and not to take on activities that could be dangerous to them (like walking too far).

A persons weakness and fatigue could be a result of some or all of the following:

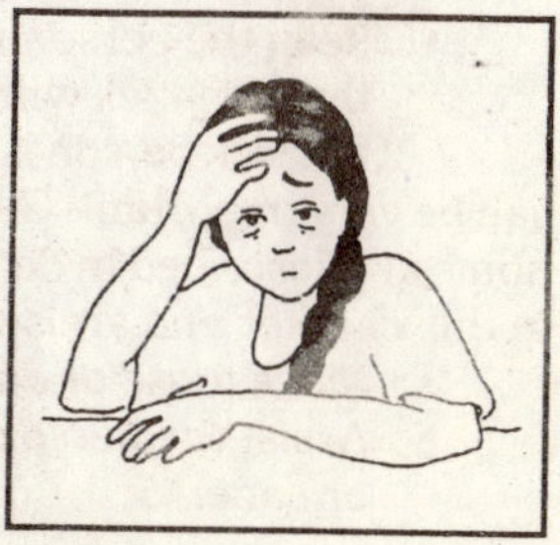

- HIV infection or HIV-related illnesses (particularly respiratory illnesses)
- poor nutrition
- depression
- anaemia.

What to do at home

If no treatable infection or other problem is found, it is important for people to learn how to adjust to their limited ability. The following advice may help a person to do this:

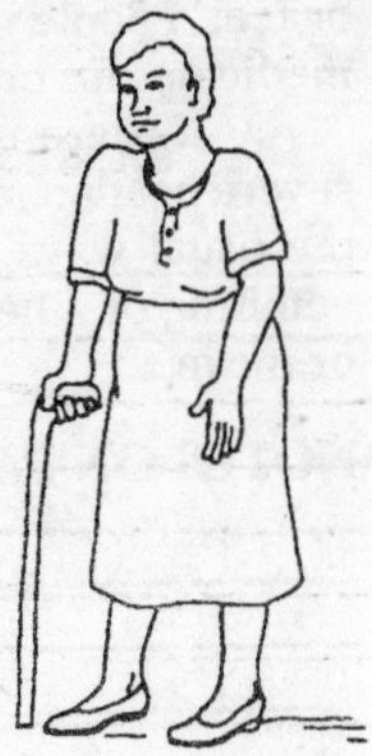

- See what can and cannot be done unaided. It can help a family to know when and for what things someone needs assistance, and help them to understand that there are still some things the sick person can do in the home, while other tasks may have to be given to others.
- Rest should be taken as often as needed.
- Help should be asked for, and accepted, from others. People will usually appreciate being told how they can help rather than having to guess and feel uncertain.
- Ways should be found of making some activities easier - for example, sitting rather than standing to bathe or cook; using a bedpan or suitable container rather than going to the toilet or latrine; using a walker, cane or wheelchair.

If someone cannot get out of bed at all they will clearly need help - see the section on skin problems in this chapter for information on the prevention of bedsores and skin problems due to prolonged inactivity. The person helping should be advised to:

- move the sick persons arms and legs gently, several, times a day
- provide a bedpan or suitable container every few hours, or more often if needed, to allow the person to empty their bowels or bladder

When someone is caring for a person with AIDS who is tired and weak they should:

- help with the persons daily needs, such as bathing, going to the toilet or latrine, getting in and out of bed, changing position in bed, eating and drinking
- keep the person involved, even if he or she is very weak, in the activities within the home.

If the sick person is weak but moving about, safety precautions can be very important. General safety precautions to be taken in the home are described in detail in the section on mental confusion later in this chapter and are summarized here as follows:

- Move loose or dangerous objects out of the way.
- Assist the person when walking or provide a walking stick or cane.

- Try not to leave the person alone for long periods.

When sick people and their families must seek help

If the sick person suddenly becomes very weak (for example, unable to walk), particularly if there are also other symptoms such as a high fever, headache or confusion.

NOTES ON TIREDNESS AND WEAKNESS

MENTAL CONFUSION AND DEMENTIA

Problems and possible causes

Some degree of mental confusion (or dementia) is common among people with AIDS. These symptoms may be caused by infection of the brain with HIV. The mental changes resulting from this may be barely noticeable or they may become a serious disability.

People with AIDS may describe feeling 'dulled" or "slow" in their thinking. It is usually the family who are the first to notice the changes.

These problems often start in a mild, barely noticeable way but may gradually worsen over time. It is not possible to predict whether the symptoms will become severe.

The mental changes may include difficulty in one or all of three areas:

- The ability to think clearly. This may be noticed as a problem in concentrating, and losing track of conversations or tasks.
- Behaviour. The person may become irritable, disinterested or unpredictable.
- Strength or coordination. The person may start dropping things more often, falling, or may develop slowness in movements, or shakiness.

HIV infection of the brain is the most common cause of mental confusion in people with AIDS. However, other possible causes include:

- the side-effects of many medicines
- infection with numerous other bacteria, viruses and parasites
- severe depression.

What to do at home

Mental confusion can be a very upsetting and frightening problem for everyone involved. People with these problems may have moments when they realize that they are not able to think as clearly as before and will be aware of actions they have taken that were inappropriate. This is deeply distressing to them. Family members are also often very upset and not sure what to do. Support and guidance from religious leaders, counsellors and friends will be very important.

There is no specific treatment for these problems and people must learn to live with them and to make the sick persons environment as safe as possible. Mental confusion in the sick person, perhaps more than any other symptom, can make care givers feel like giving up and cause them to feel overwhelmed by the demands of caring for someone they love.

A person who has a sudden change in thinking, behaviour or ability to move should seek help. Some of the sudden mental changes may be treatable and the person will recover. However, if such changes are allowed to continue, they may contribute to the rate of mental deterioration.

If it is determined that nothing further can be done, then the family will need to give whatever help they can. This will include protecting the sick person from harm.

Carers may need help to occasionally arrange time away from the home. Taking care of a sick family member for 24 hours a day, every day, is very difficult and people need physical and emotional strength to deal with this.

To prevent accidents in the home, people should:

- pay attention to open fires or boiling water
- provide canes or walkers for people who are weak or off balance when walking
- remove loose and potentially dangerous objects, including rugs
- keep walkways clear
- avoid rearranging furniture
- store poisonous or toxic substances safely out of reach
- keep medicines out of reach and only give them according to the prescribed schedule

- install handrails or put a chair in showers or tubs
- store sharp objects like knives, scissors, razors and saws safely and out of reach
- try not to leave the sick person alone and unattended for long periods.

To help the functioning of the confused or demented person, people can:

- remind the person where he or she is and what time it is - use cues to help, for example:
  - — provide reminders of daily activities in a form the person understands
  - — provide familiar objects in easily visible places, such as pictures, clocks, calendars, etc.
- keep a calm, accepting and open manner when dealing with the person
- be aware of their actions and consciously slow down and relax
- speak slowly
- use a low-pitched tone of voice this is reassuring
- ask questions that can be answered "yes" or "no"
- give simple, short directions, or explanations to questions
- be concrete and specific
- give the person lots of time to respond to questions, directions or conversation
- try to interpret the feelings the person is trying to express rather than just the words
- talk about the distant past - the persons memory of events that happened long ago may be good and this will be pleasurable.

People should avoid:

- arguing, as it will not convince the person and may only upset him or her
- directly challenging the sick persons delusions or fantasies; it is better to cast doubt in a kindly way
- giving the person multiple tasks; instead give the-person one thing at a time to do
- talking to the person as if he or she is a child
- giving choices, as this can be confusing.

To help a confused person who is upset or angry

Distraction is helpful; for example people can:

- change the subject
- provide music or switch on the radio
- give the person a manual task, e.g. folding clothes

- Ieave the room for a few minutes; the person may forget why he or she is angry
- remove the person from an upsetting situation.

The following may also help:

- maintaining a quiet environment
- setting limits
- saying "no" gently, but firmly
- not challenging or responding to the content of the angry words directed at the care giver or others.

When sick people and their families must seek help

If there is any sudden change in the persons ability to think or move, especially if this is associated with new fever, high fever, headache or difficulty in breathing.

If other mental or character changes occur - such changes should be evaluated by a health care worker, who may be able to offer help or provide treatment for the underlying cause.

A confused and aggressive person can be very difficult to manage at home. There may come a time when the people around them cannot manage and they will need the help of a health care worker in placing the person elsewhere in order to protect the sick person or family members.

NOTES ON MENTAL CONFUSION AND DEMENTIA

7

Conditions that Need Special Attention in People with HIV Infection

This chapter provides information on two conditions in people infected with HIV, tuberculosis and pregnancy, for which home care alone is not enough.
You should advise people with HIV infection, including those who have AIDS, that they should seek help from a health care worker if they think they also have tuberculosis, or if they have already become pregnant.
Again the advice is presented in a way that is designed to help you to advise an adult with AIDS or the family using the same headings as in Chapter 6.

TUBERCULOSIS

Problems and possible causes

Tuberculosis is a chronic (long-lasting), *contagious* disease that is caused by a bacterial infection. It can be cured with the correct treatment. It most often strikes young adults (15-35 years old), especially those who are weak, poorly nourished, or who live with someone who has the disease.

Tuberculosis usually affects the lungs and causes coughing. When it is severe people may cough up blood. Especially in children, young people and those with HIV infection, tuberculosis can also affect the bones, brain, lymph nodes and other parts of the body. The symptoms of tuberculosis can appear in many different ways, as indicated below:

In the South-East Asia Region, by the time most people reach adulthood, they would have been infected by the bacterium that causes tuberculosis *(Mycobacterium tuberculosis)*. However, if they are healthy, their bodys defences - the immune system - will have prevented the bacteria from causing tuberculosis. In this case people arc usually unaware that the tuberculosis bacteria are in their body, and they feel well.

The relationship between tuberculosis and HIV can be summarized in the following way:

If someone has HIV infection they are more likely to get tuberculosis

The damage to the immune system caused by HIV means the immune defences are weakened and that they can no longer keep the tuberculosis bacteria from making a person ill. The tuberculosis bacteria, which have remained quiet in the body for years in some people, now cause the disease called tuberculosis.

If someone has HIV infection the symptoms of tuberculosis can be usual or unusual

In communities where tuberculosis is very common, most people can readily recognize the disease. The most common symptoms include:

- chronic cough (lasting more than three weeks), which is often worse just after waking up, and may involve coughing up blood
- loss of weight and increasing weakness
- mild fever
- sweating at night
- pain in the upper back or chest
- loss of appetite.

If someone has AIDS, they may also develop less usual tuberculosis symptoms, such as fever without a cough. Tuberculosis can also infect the lymph nodes, especially in children - most often those in the area of the neck and shoulders. These infected nodes may become large lumps under the skin which open and drain pus, close for a time, and open and drain again.

Tuberculosis should be suspected if someone has AIDS and has respiratory or chest symptoms.

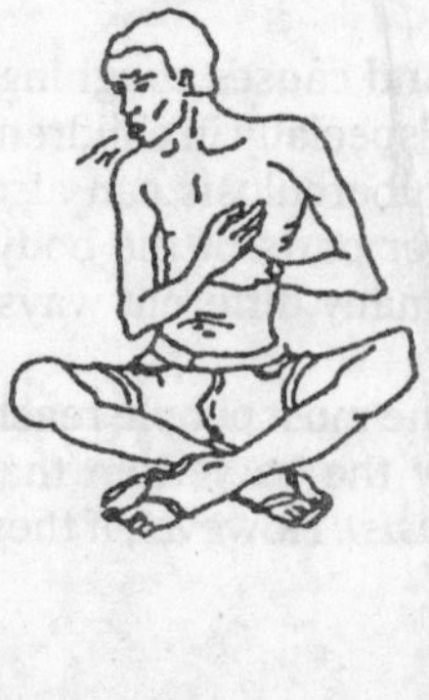

Because the possibility of having tuberculosis is so high if a person has AIDS, all people with AIDS and respiratory, chest or general symptoms that do not go away within three weeks should go to a health care worker to be tested for tuberculosis. This is particularly true if someone lives in an area where tuberculosis is common.

As tuberculosis is treatable with medicines, is highly dangerous if not treated, and can be passed on to others, it is important for people to get a prompt diagnosis through a sputum examination and/or a chest x-ray.

HIV infection and AIDS should be considered in every person with tuberculosis

Because tuberculosis and AIDS have been shown to accompany each other very often, in many areas of the world it is possible that if someone has tuberculosis they are also infected with HIV. People with tuberculosis should consider asking their health care worker to test them for HIV if this has not already been suggested.

What to do at home

Tuberculosis prevention

As a first step people should be advised to follow the principles for preventing tuberculosis which are presented in the following box.

SOME PRINCIPLES FOR PREVENTING TUBERCULOSIS

- Everyone - without exception — should seek early assessment and health care if coughing for three weeks or more.
- Everyone - without exception "should cover their mouth when coughing.
- Everyone without exception — should spit into a closed container, not on the ground. The contents should be thrown into a fire or covered with mud.
- Everyone - without exception — should avoid being in an unventilated space with a person who has been coughing for more than three weeks.
- All homes, health facilities, workplaces and other places where people meet he ventilated - make sure there is a way in and out for fresh air.

In addition, all newborn babies and young children should be immunized against tuberculosis with BCG vaccine. This may cause a spot or slight wound at the point of injection which will usually heal in some months without any treatment. The vaccine gives good protection against the serious childhood forms of the disease. However, if a child is ill at birth or has clinical symptoms of AIDS (see Chapter 4), it should not receive BCG vaccine.

Tuberculosis is contagious, particularly when there is prolonged contact with a person with the disease. Those people - and especially children - who live in the same house with someone who has tuberculosis run a risk of becoming infected. To prevent tuberculosis from spreading to others, the whole family should be asked if they have a cough and should have their sputum tested for tuberculosis at the health centre, if necessary.

Tuberculosis treatment

There are many effective treatments available to cure tuberculosis (see Chapter 8). Treatment always includes at least two different medicines. If only one is used, the tuberculosis bacteria may become resistant (insensitive) to it. Treatment stopped too early is dangerous to both the individual and the community because this too can lead to the development of tuberculosis bacteria that are resistant to drugs. Drug-resistant tuberculosis is much more difficult and expensive to cure. Therefore, it is vitally important to ensure that people take *all* the medicines they are given for the treatment of tuberculosis, and that they complete the full course. Such medicines, if taken properly, will prevent this infection from spreading among people who live or work together.

In some countries, treatment for tuberculosis is nearly always started in a clinic or hospital and few people are treated at home. This is because of the type of medicines used and because of the need to be absolutely certain that individuals take their medicines.

Before leaving the clinic or hospital, people should be instructed on how to take the medicines at home, and should be encouraged to ask for clear instructions. When a person returns home, they should have enough anti-tuberculosis medicines to last for about one month or at least until their next scheduled clinic appointment. After returning home from the clinic or hospital, people should be seen by a health care worker and be given a new supply of medicines every month.

It is very important that the medicines are taken regularly, exactly as prescribed. People taking anti-tuberculosis medication will begin to feel better but must still take their medication until the course is completed, otherwise symptoms will reappear and they will again become infectious to their family. Family members can help patients take their medication by reminding them. This is important to the whole family and not only to the patient with tuberculosis. It can take many months to cure tuberculosis completely. Nobody should ever stop taking their medicines, even if they feel better, *unless* instructed to do so by a health care worker.

Anti-tuberculosis medicines are also expensive. Most governments have programmes that provide them free or at reduced cost. If people are finding it difficult to afford the cost, they may be able to get help through the nongovernmental assistance agencies.

IMPORTANT

Be sure that people with tuberculosis know:

- Which medicines they must take to cure tuberculosis
- how to take the medicines
- for how long they need to take them
- what side-effects they should watch for
- that they should not stop treatment when they feel better
- that prompt, complete treatment will cure tuberculosis
- that prompt, complete treatment is the best way to prevent further spread

Women should know that they should avoid pregnancy while on treatment as their condition may worsen after childbirth and that they may infect their newborn.

If the main problems experienced are with breathing, people should avoid the things that can make their symptoms worse, for example, anxiety, strenuous activity, smoke, dust, aerosol sprays and smoking of any type. People should also avoid lying flat, and instead should sit up or lie with their head raised. See the section on "Coughing and difficulty in breathing" in Chapter 6 for more specific information.

When sick people and their families must seek help

- If the sick person has AIDS and has a cough or other signs and symptoms that suggest they might also have tuberculosis.
- If the sick person has a reaction to the anti-tuberculosis medicines.
- If the white parts of the sick persons eyes become yellow.

NOTES ON TUBERCULOSIS

PREGNANCY AND CHILDBIRTH

Problems

If a woman has AIDS, she is likely to have problems during her pregnancy, during delivery of the baby or after the birth.

Such problems may include:

- miscarriage - loss of the baby during pregnancy
- fevers and infections
- premature labour - delivery occurring earlier than it should, often causing the death of the baby
- a smaller baby - the weight at birth of even a full-term baby can be much lower than normal; babies with a low birth weight are more likely to have subsequent problems
- infections after birth - these are much more common in women with AIDS and can be life-threatening; women who are HIV-positive might have severe infections after delivery (puerperal sepsis) which do not respond to the usual treatment with antibiotics.

WHAT TO DO AT HOME

Antenatal care

All pregnant women should receive antenatal care during pregnancy. This is more important if they have AIDS. Women infected with HIV should be advised to follow the routine recommendations for all pregnant women. These are:

- A health care worker (trained birth attendant, nurse/midwife, doctor) should be contacted as soon as the pregnancy is suspected so that care can be started as early as possible.
- No medicines should be taken except those prescribed by a health care worker (women should always tell their health care worker that they arc pregnant if they see them for another reason). Some medicines can be harmful to both the mother and her developing baby so it is best not to take any risks.
- The mother should eat for herself and for her growing child. She should eat from the three main groups of foods described in the section on nutrition problems in Chapter 6.
- Iron and folic acid should be taken daily. (You can get these tablets from your health worker/health centre.) This is important as it will prevent anaemia in both the mother and child. Anaemia causes complications such as heavy bleeding after childbirth.

- Rest should be taken for one hour at least in the afternoon. This is important for the baby's growth.
- If possible, heavy weights should not be lifted and heavy work should be avoided. This may lead to premature labour and make one feel easily tired.
- One should keep clean by bathing daily. Other practices for avoiding infection mentioned in Chapter 3 should be followed.
- If possible, it is better to avoid sexual intercourse. If this is not possible, then safer sex should be practised throughout pregnancy. It will protect the mother and the baby from other infections.
- The health centre/clinic should be visited three times at least during the pregnancy for check-up to see whether the mother is alright and the baby is growing properly.
- Pregnant mothers should ensure that they are properly immunized against tetanus to protect themselves and the baby (two doses if you have not been immunized earlier and one dose if immunized within the past five years) .

Before delivery

You may recommend that the mother plan to deliver in a health centre or hospital. If this is not possible, and there are no complications, then people, with the help of a health care worker, should prepare for delivery in the home so that it poses the least risk to the mother, the baby, and those who help with the delivery.

- Advise people to prepare beforehand the things which they will need for a safe delivery.
- A separate room or part of the room should be identified where the delivery has to take place. The place should be kept clean and warm.
- If possible, a disposable delivery kit should be procured from the health centre or from the market for use during delivery. Use of a disposable delivery kit is important for prevention of tetanus and other infections in the newborn and in the mother. The disposable delivery kit should contain a piece of soap for washing the hands of the birth attendant and for washing the genitalia of the woman, a razor blade for cutting the cord, two nail sticks for cleaning the nails of the birth attendant, two gauze pieces for drying the cord stump, two cotton swabs for cleaning the eyes of the baby and three cord ties for tying the cord. If a disposable delivery kit is not available, then the following should be arranged:
  - — two clean thick threads for tying the umbilical cord
  - — one clean new razor blade for cutting the cord
  - — soap

In addition, the following should be kept ready:

- several large pieces of cloth for wiping and wrapping the baby (about 1 metre by 1.5 metres each)
- one metre plastic sheet or old cloth to put under the mother
- one container of antiseptic solution such as iodine solution or gentian violet
- cotton wool or clean cloths for applying antiseptic solution to the cord stump
- gloves or plastic bags for the delivery assistant and for handling the afterbirth
- one container of clean (boiled and cooled) water for cleaning the mother, the baby and the assistants hands and arms
- pads for the vaginal area of the mother to catch drainage following the birth these can be made from pieces of old but clean cotton cloth
- warm clean clothing for the baby following birth
- clean clothing for the mother to change into after the delivery
- a packet of household bleaching powder
- a bucket for making the bleach solution.

Care during childbirth

As the labour pains start, the trained birth attendant or health worker who has been looking after the mother should be contacted.

- If a safe delivery kit is not available, the birth attendant should boil as many items as possible in the list given above, especially those used for cutting, tying and wiping the cord stump.
- The mother should lie on the piece of cloth or plastic sheet.
- The birth attendant or helper should make the bleach solution by mixing one level teaspoonful of bleaching powder per litre of clean water.
- The trained helper should wash her hands thoroughly with soap and water (after removing her rings and bangles).
- Any would or abrasion on the hands of the birth attendant should be covered with a watertight dressing.
- The birth attendant should not do unnecessary vaginal examinations. This will protect the mother from infections as well as decrease the birth attendant's exposure to HIV.
- The birth attendant should wear clean sterile gloves (clean kitchen gloves washed with soap and warm water if regular latex gloves are not available) or cover the hands with clean plastic cover while conducting the delivery to avoid skin contact with blood and fluid that comes out of the mother's womb. It will be ideal to wear a plastic apron also.
- The birth attendant should protect the mouth nose and eyes if possible against splashes of blood and other body fluids.

This can be done by tying a piece of cloth over their mouth and nose.

- The mother's genital area should be washed before the delivery.
- As soon as the baby is born, the attendant should clean the mouth and nose of the baby with a clean piece of cloth. A mucous extractor with a trap should be used with those babies in whom mucous suction is required.
- The umbilical cord should be tied in two places with the sterile thread and cut between the two threads with a new or sterile blade.
- The baby should be wiped dry with a clean cloth and covered with another clean cloth making sure the head and feet are covered.
- Keep the room warm and keep the baby in close contact with the mother.
- The mother's genital area should be cleaned and pads made out of clean cloth should be used.
- The mother's clothes should be changed.
- Hands should be washed thoroughly with soap and water immediately after contact with blood or other body fluids.
- The baby should be put to breast as early as possible.
- The blood-soaked cloths and placenta should be burned or buried in places where they are not likely to be dug up.
- Any blood which is spilt should be immediately cleaned with an absorbent material. The material should be soaked in bleach solution for 20 minutes and then washed.
- Clothes soiled with blood or other body fluids should be soaked in bleach solution for 20 minutes and then washed in hot soapy water.

Care after childbirth

- The mother should bathe daily and keep clean. The genital area should be washed with soap and water twice daily. The genital pads should be changed everyday, and the frequency of changing depends on the amount of bleeding. Dirty pads can lead to infections of the womb.
- The pads should be kept in a separate bag and disposed of by being burnt or thrown into a pit latrine. If the pads are to be reused, they should be soaked in household bleach solution, prepared as described earlier. The pads should be soaked for an hour in the solution and then washed with soap and hot water.
- Safer sex should be practised. Correct and consistent use of condoms is important not only to prevent a pregnancy, but also to protect from other infections.

- More of regular food should be eaten to get back the strength after the pregnancy and childbirth. Plenty of fluids should be taken.

When women and their families must seek help

During pregnancy help should be sought immediately if any of th following happens:

- bleeding from the vagina
- swelling of the feet and headaches
- sharp pain in the abdomen
- the bag of waters breaks
- convulsions
- baby stops moving

At the time of childbirth or immediately after childbirth help should be sought if any of the following happens:

- severe bleeding from the vagina
- labour pains do not progress satisfactorily
- a part of the body other than the baby's head comes out first, e.g. breech, cord etc.
- convulsions
- the placenta does not come out
- baby has difficultly in breathing
- baby does not breathe or cry soon after birth

After childbirth help should be sought if any of the following happens to the mother:

- severe bleeding from the vagina
- fever
- foul-smelling vaginal discharge
- severe abdominal pain
- painful breasts
- breast-feeding problems
- convulsions.

In the baby:

- high fever
- convulsions
- yellowness
- pus coming out of the umbilical stump
- difficulty in breathing
- feeding poorly

NOTES ON PREGNANCY AND CHILDBIRTH

8

General Informatior. on the use of Medicines

People seeking a cure for AIDS may spend a lot of money on medicines from shops, health care workers and traditional healers. Unfortunately much of this money is wasted because such medicines are not effective, may cause other problems, and use up money that would be much better spent on food, clothing, or other essential items for all the family.

This chapter provides the information you need in order to teach people how to use medicines safely and effectively. It also provides a brief description of the medicines commonly used to treat symptoms that occur in people with AIDS.

Please note that not all the medicines listed in this guide are needed in a medicine kit or in the home. Because different medicines are available in different countries, information has sometimes been given on a number of medicines that do the same job. It is wise to:

Keep and use only a small number of medicines.

(It is best to use familiar medicines that you understand well.)

Teaching notes on the use of medicines

It is essential that anyone taking medicines (whether prescribed or bought from a shop) follows the instructions for their safe and effective use. Medicines not taken according to instructions can be useless or even harmful, causing further illness. It can be very confusing for a person and their family when they are provided with several different medicines, all with different instructions. You must make sure that your patients and their families know how to take the medicines you recommend.

There is some danger in the use of any medicine.

Whenever you recommend a medicine, it is a good idea to give the patient and the family written instructions. This can be useful to anyone involved with the care of a sick person. Someone can usually be found to read it. You should explain the instructions and ask the patient or members of the family to repeat them to you. Make sure they understand. Below is an example of a written schedule.

WRITTEN MEDICINE SCHEDULE

Name of medicine	*Purpose*	*Description*	*When to give*	*Comments*
Aspirin or paracetamol	for fever, headaches, pain	white tablet	take 1 or 2 at least every 8 hours	take with meals or after food
Calamine lotion	for itching and irritated skin	pink liquid	apply to skin as necessary	do not take by mouth

To help remind people who cannot read when to take their medicine, you can give them a note like this:

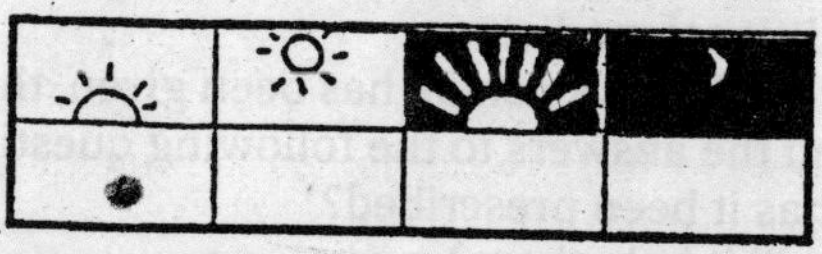

In the blanks below the pictures, draw the amount of medicine they should take and explain carefully what it means.

Here are three examples:

This means one tablet four times a day: one at sunrise, one at noon, one at sunset, and one in the middle of the night.

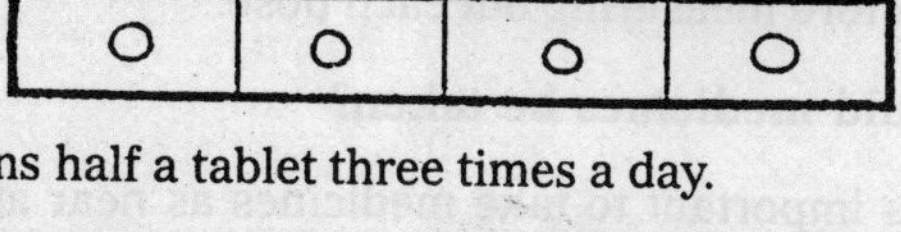

This means half a tablet three times a day.

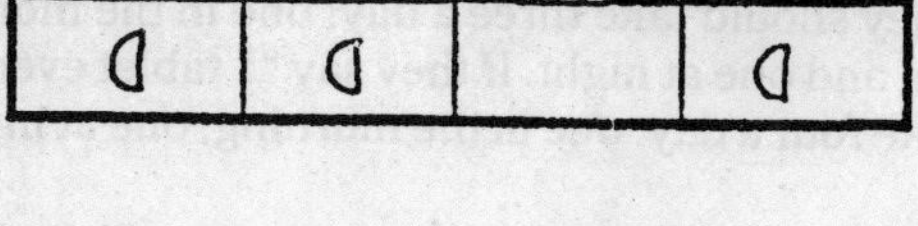

This means two teaspoonfuls twice a day.

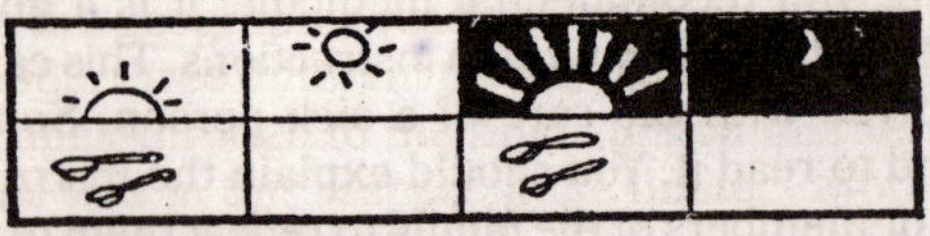

HOW TO USE MEDICINES

People may have been advised to take medicines by a health care worker or may have decided to buy their own medicines without such advice. In either case, people must know how to use medicines correctly to get the most benefit from them and to avoid any harmful effects.

How can people learn about medicines?

You, the health care worker, should give people the information they need to know. The people who sell medicines may also be helpful but remember, their primary goal is to make money through selling. Instructions about taking any medicine and the name of the medicine should be written on the container it is sold in. If a person is already taking medicine for another condition, such as a heart problem or ulcers, they should consult their doctor before taking any additional medicines.

For any medicine a person has been given, they should know and understand the answers to the following questions:

- Why has it been prescribed?
- How will it help them?
- How should it be taken?
- For how long should it be taken?
- What side-effects, if any, should they watch for?

The ability to use medicines correctly is very important for health and safety. All labels should be checked by the person before they leave the health centre or shop. If the label says:

- Keep cool—the medicine should be kept out of sunlight and out of damp places.
- Shake—the medicine should be shaken for a full minute before measuring out each dose.

How should medicines be taken?

It is important to take medicines as near as possible to the time recommended. Some medicines should be taken only once a day, but others must be taken more often. If the person does not have a clock, it does not matter. If the directions say "1 tablet every 8 hours", they should take three a day: one in the morning, one in the afternoon, and one at night. If they say "1 tablet every 6 hours", they should take four a day: one in the morning, one at midday, one in the afternoon, and one at night. Before they leave the health centre or the shop with the medicine they must be sure they understand how often to take it. If the directions say:

- On an empty stomach the medicine should be taken at least one hour after a meal, or 30 minutes before a meal.
- With meals this can also mean with snacks. People should make sure that they have eaten something before taking the medicine.

If vomiting occurs within 20 minutes after taking the medicine, the dose should be repeated.

Advice for people who are giving medicines to children

- Liquid medicines can be squirted slowly into the side of the childs mouth with a dropper or syringe, or poured from a spoon.
- Always praise a child after he or she has taken medicine.
- If the medicine tastes bad, tell the child so in advance.
- If a pill cannot be swallowed, crush it and mix it with the smallest amount possible of something the child likes to eat. However, do not "hide" the medicine in food or the child may begin to refuse food.
- If the child vomits immediately after taking a medicine, give the dose again. But if vomiting occurs 20 or more minutes after taking the medicine, do not repeat the dose.

Medicines to be used with caution in people with AIDS

There are certain medicines that can have more side-effects, or can cause more problems, in people with AIDS. People should be aware of which these are so that they can watch for any reactions they might have to them. They include medicines commonly given to treat infections, and medicines that are used only rarely:

- sulfonamides
- steroids.

Steroids (such as cortisone and hydrocortisone) deserve special mention. These medicines suppress the immune system and so they are particularly dangerous for people with AIDS because their immune system is already weakened by the disease. Steroids worsen the problems that come with AIDS by reducing even further the body's ability to fight off common infections. People with AIDS should only take steroids after very serious consideration by a medical doctor. They should only take them as part of the treatment for another problem.

Which medicines should people use?

The next section describes the medicines that might be used

at home for treating the symptoms that can develop in people with AIDS. They are grouped here according to the symptoms they are used to treat. For example, medicines used to treat pain are listed under the heading, "Medicines for pain". The symptoms themselves and how they can be treated at home are described in Chapters 6 and 7.

MEDICINES COMMONLY USED TO TREAT SYMPTOMS IN PEOPLE WITH AIDS

Medicines in this section are listed under each heading according to their *generic names* (scientific names) rather than their *brand names* (the names given by the manufacturers). Medicines are described under the following symptoms:

Medicines for infections

- antibiotics

Medicines for fever:

- aspirin
- paracetamol

Medicines for diarrhoea:

- Acute
  - — oral rehydration salts
- Persistent

Medicines for skin problems:

- General
  - — calamine lotion
- Bacterial infections
  - — gentian violet
  - — potassium permanganate
  - — hydrogen peroxide
- Yeast infections (oral and vaginal)
  - — gentian violet
  - — potassium permanganate
  - — nystatin
  - — clotrimazole
  - — ketoconazole
- Scabies
  - — benzyl benzoate

Medicines for nutrition problems:

- vitamin and mineral supplements

Medicines for nausea and vomiting:

- anti-emetics

Medicines for pain:

- aspirin
- paracetamol
- narcotic pain killers

Medicines for tuberculosis:

- isoniazid
- ethambutol
- rifampicin
- pyrazinamide

Medicines for infections

Antibiotics a general guide

Almost every person with AIDS will be given an antibiotic at some point during his or her illness to fight an infection.

When used correctly antibiotics are extremely useful and important medicines. They fight certain infections and diseases caused by bacteria. Well-known antibiotics are *penicillin, tetracycline, cotrimoxzole* and *chloramphenicol.* The *sulfonamides* have a similar effect and are also considered here. It should be noted that medicines containing sulfonamides can cause severe allergic reactions in people with AIDS, such as unusual itching or widespread rashes.

Different antibiotics work in different ways against specific infections. All antibiotics have dangers in their use, but some are far more dangerous than others. Great care must be taken in the choice and use of antibiotics:

- People should never take an antibiotic unless it has been prescribed by a health care worker for a specific reason. Left-over antibiotics should not be used to treat a new infection.
- People must continue to use the antibiotics they have been prescribed for the full length of time they are told. Some illnesses, like tuberculosis, need to be treated for many months or years after the person feels better.
- If the antibiotic causes a skin rash, itching, difficulty in breathing, or any other reaction, people should stop using it and immediately contact a health care worker. If these reactions do occur people should always mention this to the health care worker who prescribes medicine for them.

People should be encouraged to remember the name of any medicine they have a bad reaction to, so that they can tell a health care worker in the future.

- The antibiotic should only be used at the recommended dose - no more, no less. You should explain to people that the dose depends on the illness and on their age or weight, and that increasing or decreasing the dose can be harmful, or can make the medicine useless.
- Antibiotics can kill bacteria. However, not all bacteria are harmful and antibiotics often kill good bacteria along with the harmful ones. For example, people with AIDS given antibiotics often develop fungal infections of the mouth (thrush - see the section on "Mouth and throat problems" in Chapter 6), skin or vagina (see the section on 'Genital problems" in Chapter 6). This is because the antibiotics kill the bacteria that help keep the fungus under control in the body. Similarly, certain antibiotics may lead to diarrhoea - the antibiotics kill some of the bacteria necessary for digestion, upsetting the natural balance of bacteria in the intestines.
- When antibiotics are used incorrectly, they become less effective. When attacked many times by the same antibiotic, bacteria become stronger and are no longer killed by it. They become resistant to the antibiotic. For this reason, certain diseases like tuberculosis can become more difficult to treat over time if the antibiotics for them are not used in the right way.

Medicines for fever

These include aspirin and paracetamol. The recommended doses for these medicines are given in the section on medicines for pain in this chapter.

Medicines for diarrhoea

Treatment of acute diarrhoea

Oral rehydration salts (ORS). For diarrhoea with no blood in stools, no specific medicines are needed. An oral rehydration ...n made with ORS is the best means of preventing dehydration ...g from diarrhoea. See the section on 'Diarrhoea" in Chapter ...tructions on how to prepare ORS solution.

...nt of persistent diarrhoea

...eving the symptoms of persistent diarrhoea, especially in people with AIDS, can be a difficult task. The diarrhoea does not usually have a known cause and when it begins to interfere with normal activity, eating, or is very emotionally burdensome, a health care worker may prescribe specific medicines.

Medicines for skin problems

General

Calamine lotion may be rubbed on the skin to soothe itching or irritation. It should never be taken by mouth.

Bacterial infections

Gentian violet comes as a ready-made solution or as dark blue crystals that should be mixed with clean water to make a solution. To use the crystals, it is necessary to dissolve one teaspoonful in half a litre of water. This medicine helps fight certain skin infections, and has many uses.

Potassium permanganate comes as dark red crystals. It makes a good antiseptic (bacteria-killing) solution for soaking infected sores. A pinch of the crystals should be added to one litre of clean water or one teaspoonful in a four to five-litre bucket of water for soaking infected sores.

Hydrogen peroxide comes as a liquid. It should be kept in a dark bottle, as light destroys its effect. This medicine helps to clean deeply infected wounds on the skin .

Oral yeast infections (thrush)

Before using home remedies or medicines prescribed by a health care worker, a person should try cleaning the mouth with a soft toothbrush and then rinsing with salt water or lemon juice. Next, people can use gentian violet or potassium permanganate. See the section on 'Mouth and throat problems" in Chapter 6.

The medicines most commonly prescribed by a health care worker for treatment of oral fungal infections are antifungal agents such as nystatin or clotrimazole. A solution or suspension should be held in the mouth for at least one minute and then swallowed. Lozenges should be sucked in the mouth until dissolved. It may be necessary to take these medicines three or four times a day.

In some people, the thrush involves not only the mouth but the entire oesophagus, causing pain on swallowing and a burning sensation in the chest. Treatment for this can be provided by a health care worker and includes *antifungal* medicines such as *ketoconazole,* which is taken by mouth every 12 hours for 14 days.

Vaginal yeast infections

Antifungal agents (creams or suppositories) may be prescribed to cure vaginal yeast infections. These should be used once or twice a day for 5-7 days. It may help to line underclothes with cotton cloth of some sort since the medicine will drain from the vagina.

Medicines for nutrition problems

Vitamin and mineral supplements come in many forms, but tablets are usually the cheapest and work well. Injections of vitamins are rarely necessary, are a waste of money, cause unnecessary pain, and sometimes cause abscesses. Tonics and elixirs often do not contain the most important vitamins and are usually too expensive for the good they do. Nutritious food is the best source of vitamins and minerals. If additional vitamins and minerals are needed, tablets can be used but people should make sure the tablets contain the important vitamins and minerals they need.

With standard "multivitamin" tablets (tablets that contain several different vitamins), one tablet a day is usually enough. Vitamins should be taken with, or soon after meals. In addition, pregnant women need extra amounts of iron and folic acid.

Medicines for nausea and vomiting

Round-the-clock treatment with medicines for nausea and vomiting (*anti-emetics*) may become necessary if these symptoms become a big problem. They should only be taken on the advice of a health care worker. Some have serious side-effects, for example:

- nervous system effects with trembling or inability to control the movements of the neck or eyes
- fatigue, sleepiness and possibly depression; people taking anti-emetics should therefore not drive or operate machinery.

Medicines for pain

Aspirin can be useful to reduce pain, to lower fever, and to reduce inflammation. It may also help to calm a cough and reduce itching. Aspirin usually comes in tablets of 300-500 mg and should be given to adults every eight hours (or two to three times per day). For someone suffering from severe joint pains a higher dose may be recommended.

Aspirin should not be taken by children. It should *not* be used by people who have indigestion or heartburn because it can make these problems much worse. In some people, aspirin causes stomach upsets. To avoid this, aspirin can be taken with milk, some bicarbonate of soda, a lot of water, or with meals. If ringing in the ears is experienced, this is a sign that the amount of aspirin which is being taking should be lowered. Aspirin must be kept out of the reach of children as large amounts can poison them.

Paracetamol is used for many of the same problems as aspirin, such as pain and fever. However, it is safer for children and does not cause stomach problems, such as ulcers, so it can be used instead of aspirin if such problems are experienced. Paracetamol, rather than aspirin, should be given to children. Similar precautions should also be taken to keep paracetamol out of the reach of children.

Paracetamol usually comes in tablets of 500 mg and should be given at least every eight hours (or two to three times per day) as follows:

- adults: 1 or 2 tablets (500-1000 mg)
- children 8-12 years: 1 tablet (500 mg)
- children 3-7 years: half a tablet (250 mg)
- children 6 months-2 years: quarter of a tablet (125 mg)
- babies under 6 months: one eighth of a tablet (62 mg).

Narcotic painkillers, such as codeine and morphine, may be prescribed by a health care worker and are used only for severe pain. These medicines are addictive, which means that if someone continues to take them they may need increasingly higher doses to get the same therapeutic effect, and may find that they crave for them at times when they are not having pain. Other side-effects that may be troublesome include nausea, drowsiness, constipation, depression, fatigue and itching.

Make sure that people are advised to take extra fluids to prevent constipation if they are taking such medicines. If people are taking this type of medicine make sure they follow the directions carefully and do not drive or operate machinery.

Medicines for tuberculosis

Almost all countries in the world have guidelines or standard treatment protocols which they use in the treatment of tuberculosis. You should follow your country's standard treatments. This section describes the most common medicines used in the treatment of tuberculosis. At least two medicines to treat tuberculosis should always be given at the same time. This section is meant to supplement the information given in Chapter 7 on tuberculosis and you should refer back to that section. The most important points about the treatment of tuberculosis are shown in the box below .

- *Tuberculosis is curable if medicines are taken as prescribed.*
- *If medicines are stopped early, individuals get sick again and become infectious to others.*
- *If medicines are taken as prescribed, individuals become completely non-infectious to others.*

Isoniazid comes in tablet form and should be taken before the morning meal. Tablets should be stored out of direct sunlight.

Isoniazid occasionally causes liver problems. If this happens people will notice itching and the white part of their eyes turns yellow. They should return immediately to the health care worker who prescribed this medicine. In rare cases, the medicine causes anaemia, nerve pains in the hands and feet, muscle twitching or even fits. These side-effects can usually be prevented by taking a tablet of vitamin B6 (pyridoxine) every day.

Isoniazid is usually given for a long period of time, for example six months to one year, until the tuberculosis is considered completely cured.

This medicine is safe to use during pregnancy.

Ethambutol comes in tablet form.

It may cause eye problems if taken in large doses for a long time. If people notice that their eyesight seems worse, with blurring of vision or colour bindness, they should return to the health care worker who prescribed this medicine.

It is usually given once a day for two to twelve months.

Ethambutol is not advised for use in children less than six years old.

Rifampicin comes as single tablets of 150-300 mg or in a combined form, mixed with isoniazid, as tablets that contain 150-300 mg of *rifampicin* and 100-150 mg of isoniazid.

Rifampicin should be taken on an empty stomach, at least 30 minutes before the morning meal, since food interferes with the absorption of the medicine. It should be stored out of direct sunlight and in a dry place.

Rifampicin can be used in pregnancy.

Side-effects are not very common. This medicine may cause liver problems which can cause the white part of the eye to turn yellow. If this happens the person should return immediately to the health care worker who prescribed the medicine.

Rifampicin is likely to stain urine, tears, saliva, faeces and other body fluids an orange colour. If people notice this discoloration, they should *not* stop taking the medicine, as it is a normal reaction and is completely harmless.

Occasionally the medicine may cause flushing, itching, rash, fever or flu-like symptoms. If people experience any of these problems, they should discuss them with their health care worker.

Pyrazinamide comes in tablet form and should be taken in the morning with or without food.

Pyrazinamide is safe to take during pregnancy.

The most common side-effect of this medicine is joint pains. These pains tend to occur in the shoulders and are relieved by mild pain medicines. The pain usually goes away within a short period of time. This medicine may also cause liver problems which makes the white part of the eye turn yellow. If this happens the patient should return to the health centre or hospital immediately.

Streptomycin and thiacetazone are not recommended as part of tuberculosis treatment.

NOTES ON THE USE OF MEDICINES

9

Pictures for Teaching

The Story of Ravi and Radha that was presented early in the book shows how HIV comes into a family, and what happens over several years. The story of Mod is used to show how a young man gets infected with HIV by injecting drugs. The characters are shown in the pictures to make it more interesting. These pictures are reproduced in the following section for use during teaching. The pictures can be photocopied or removed from the book to be displayed, perhaps fixed to a wall or a piece of cardboard. They can also be numbered according to the order in which you intend to use them.

You can also present these stories in the form of plays.

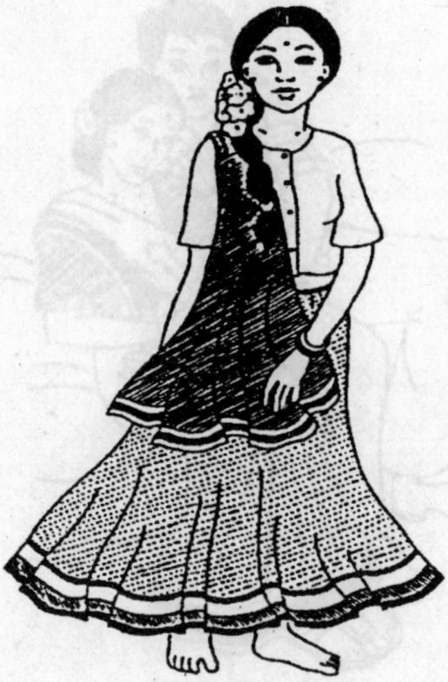

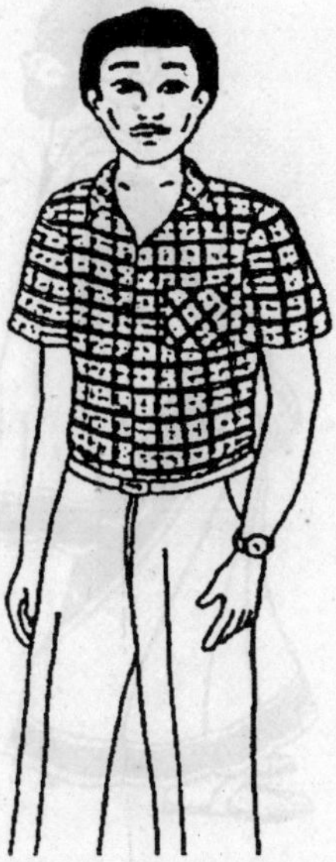

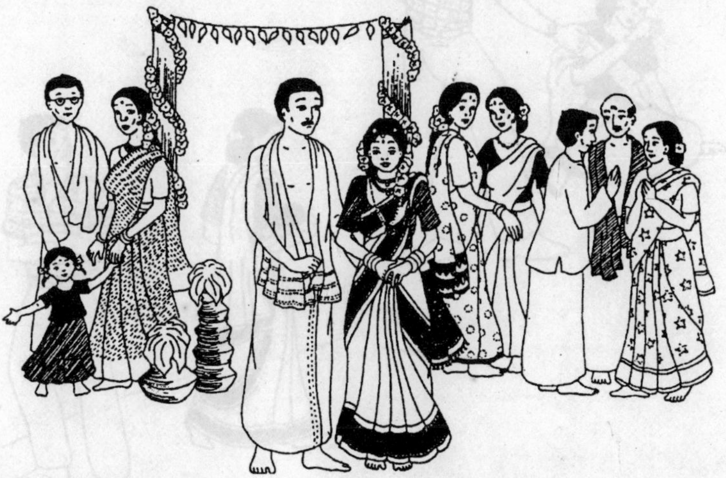

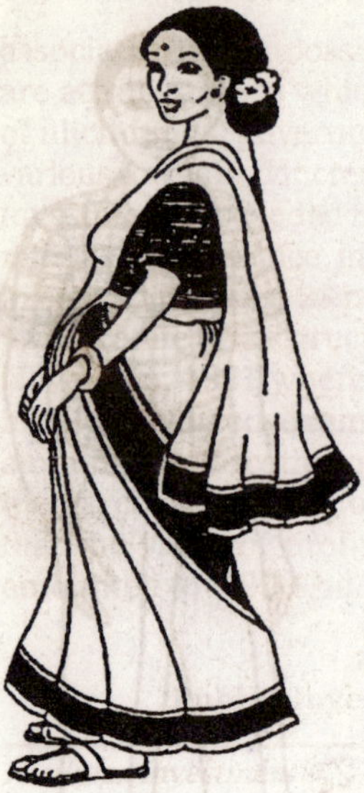

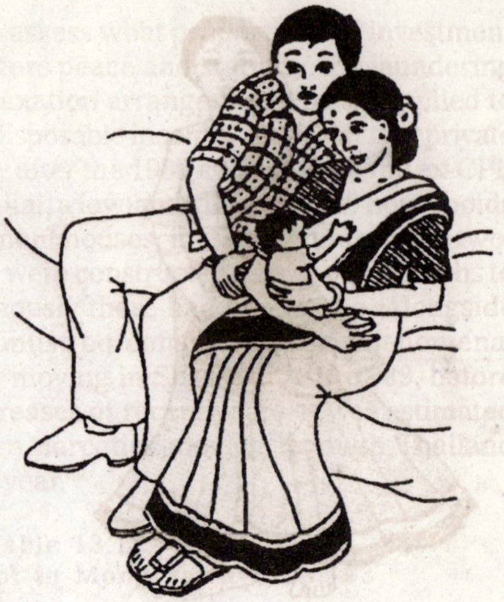

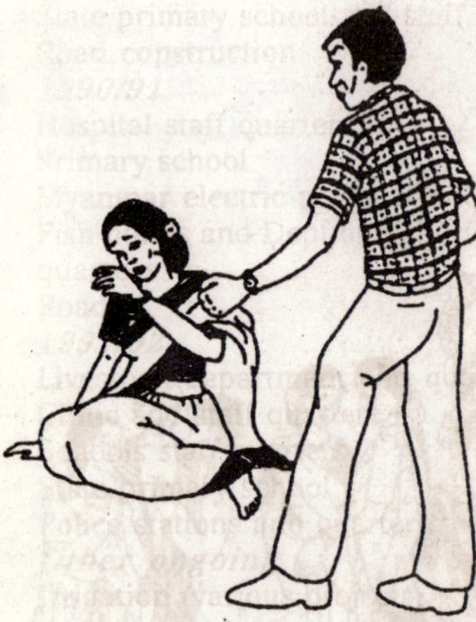

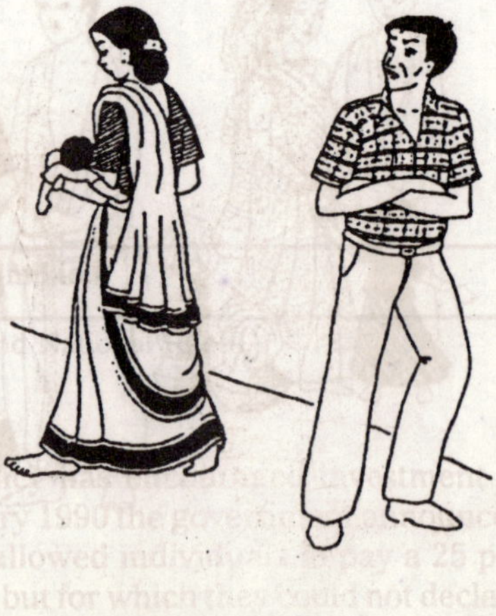

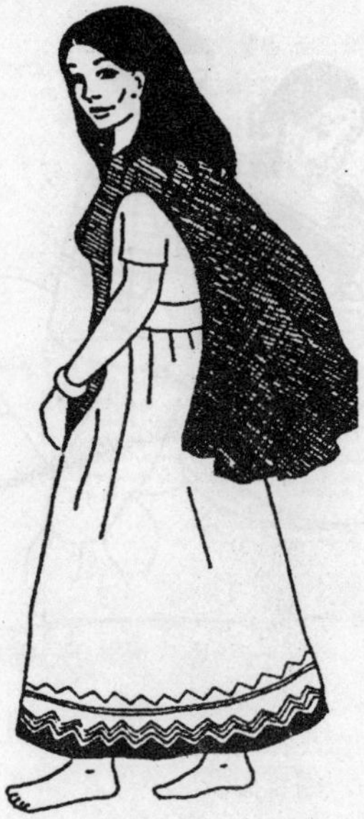

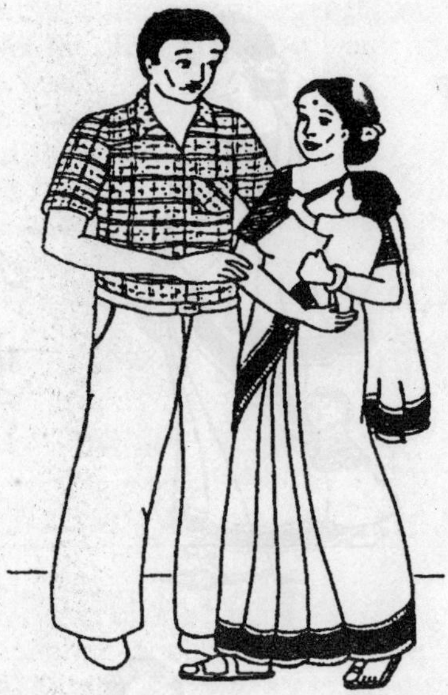

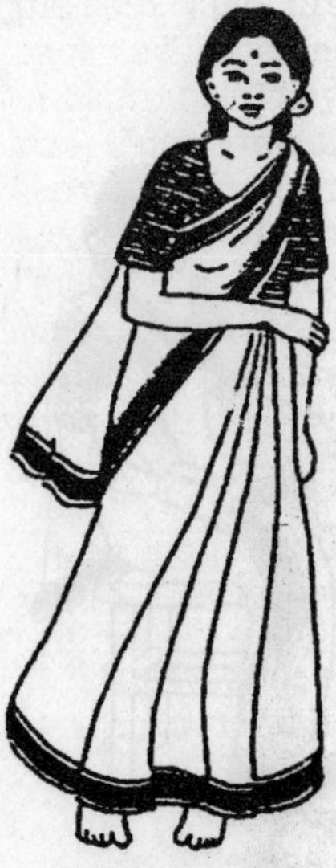

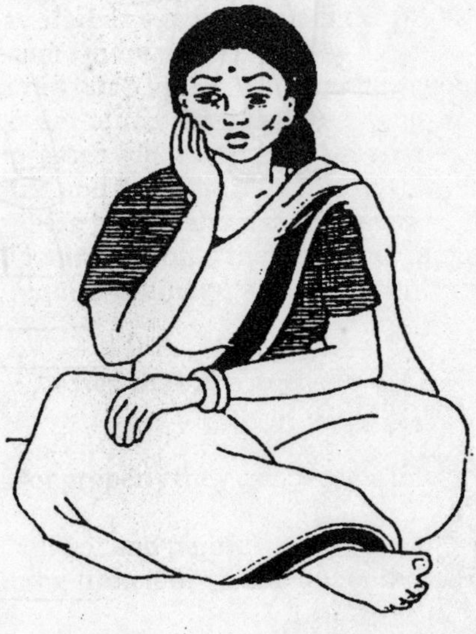

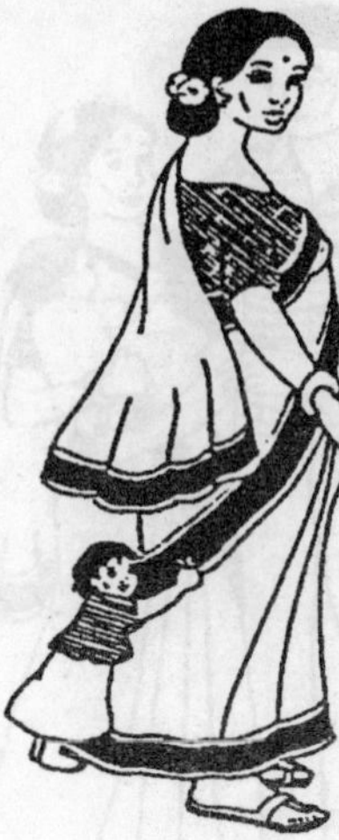

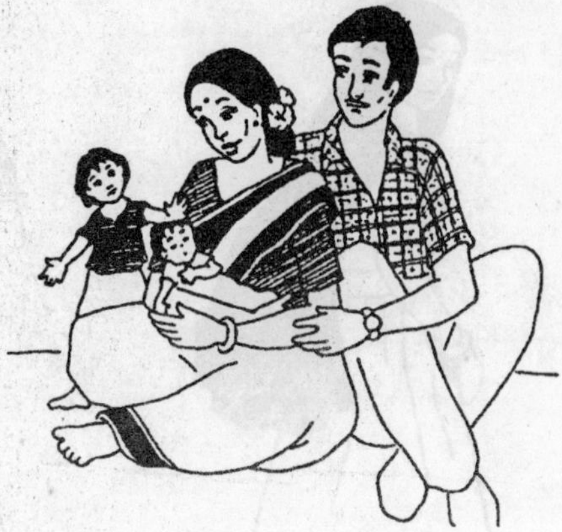

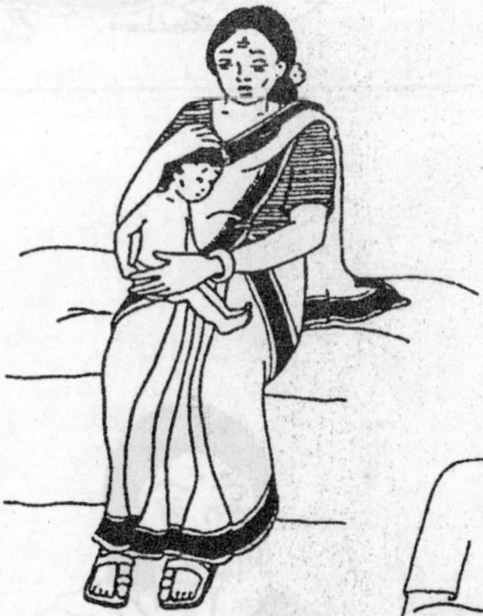

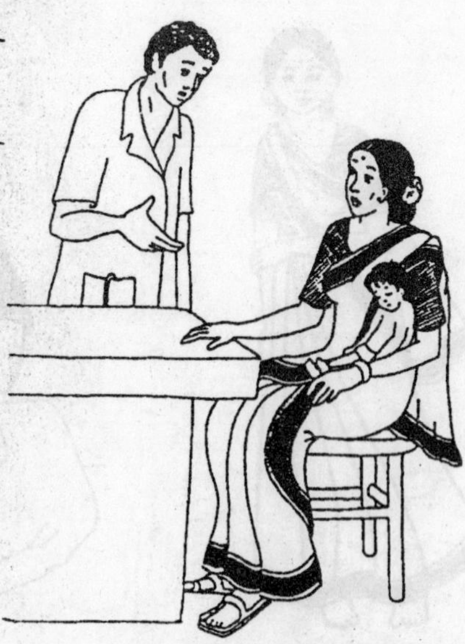

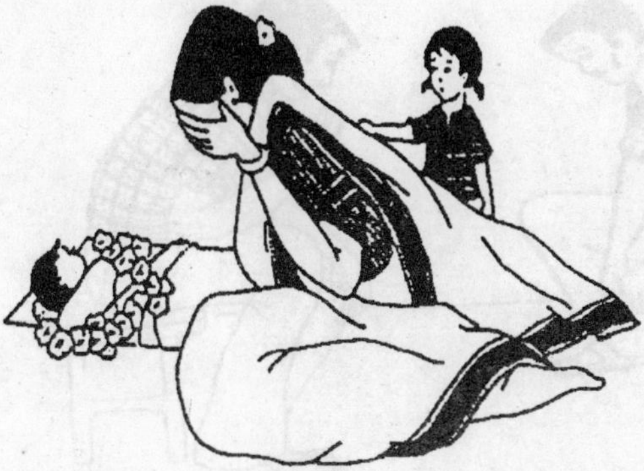

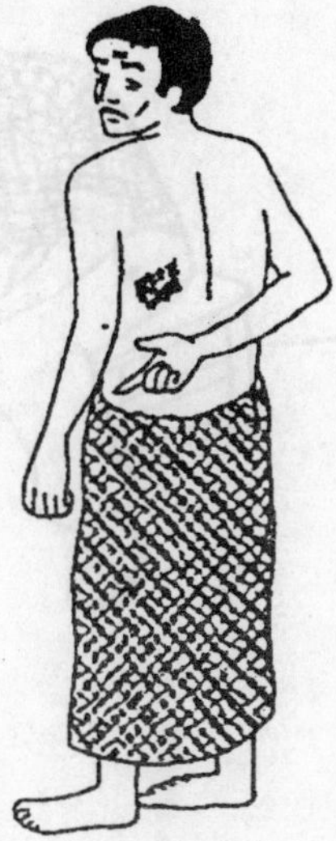

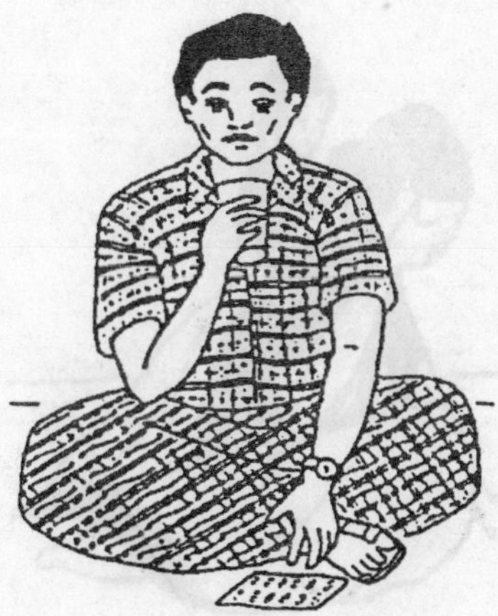

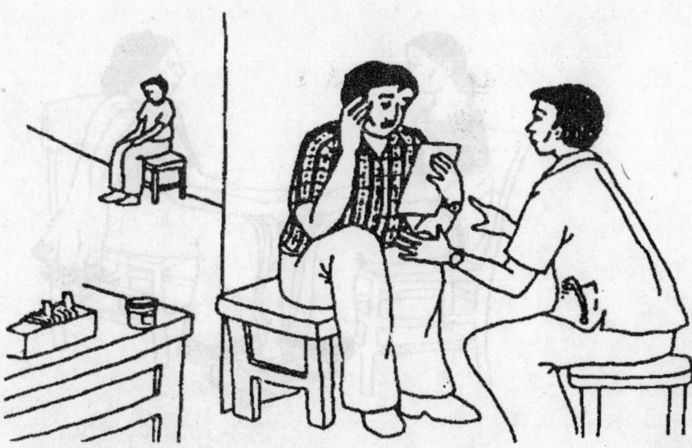

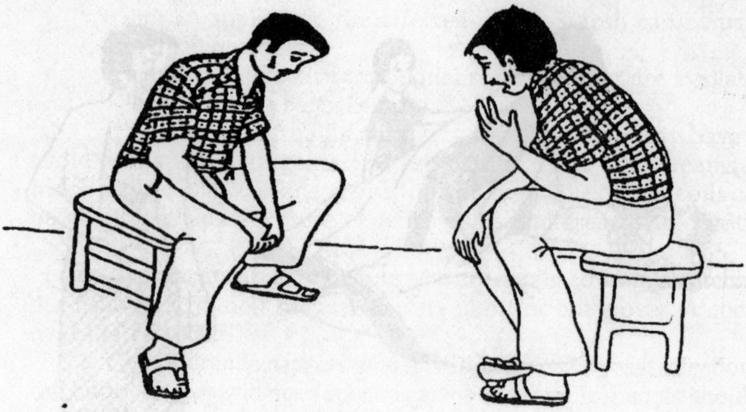

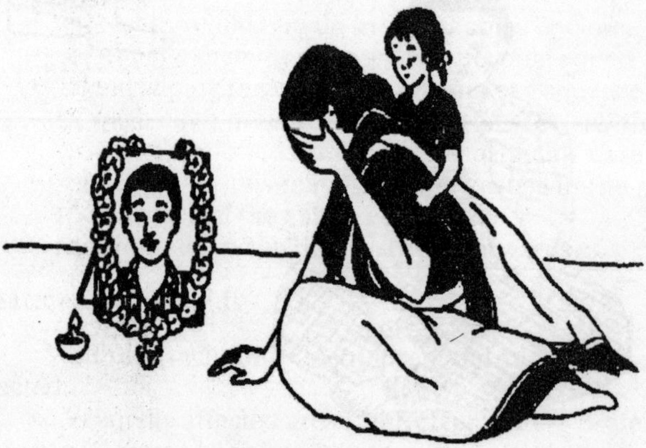

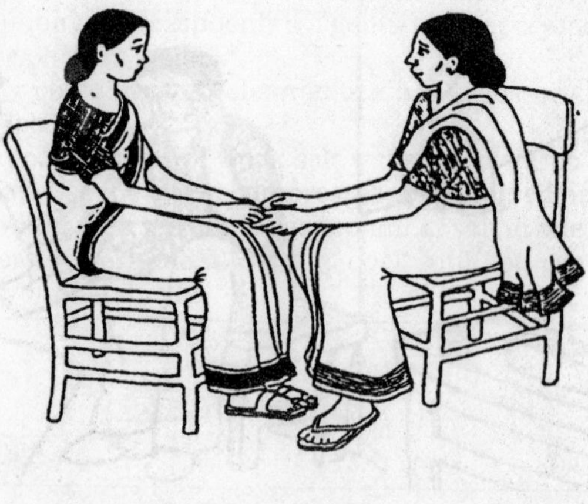

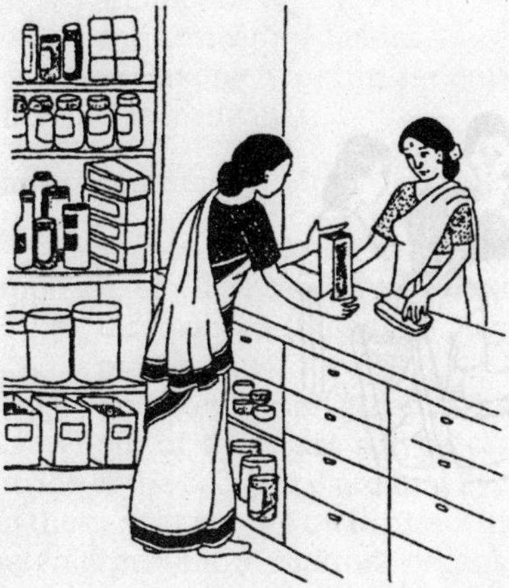

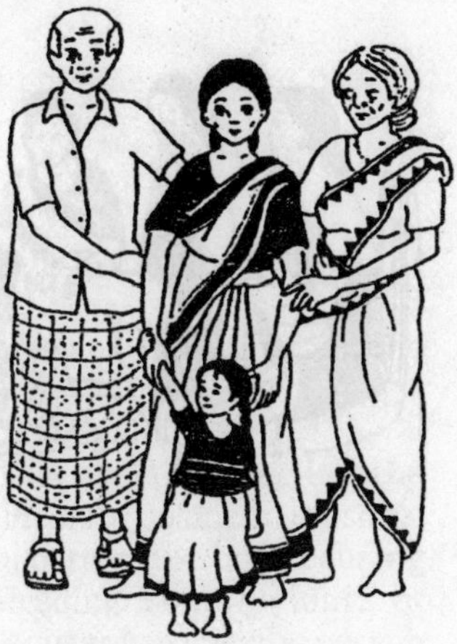

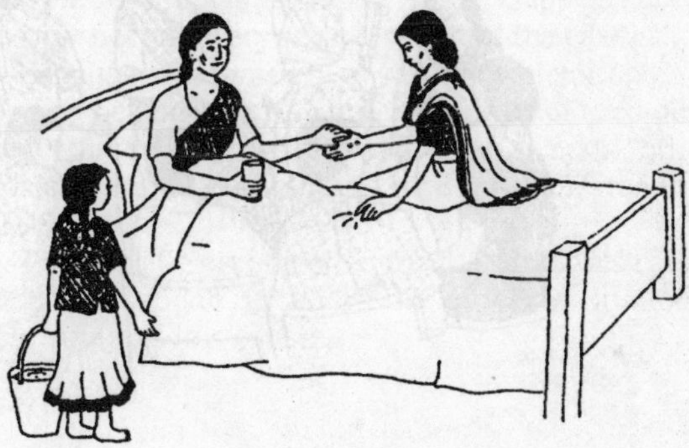

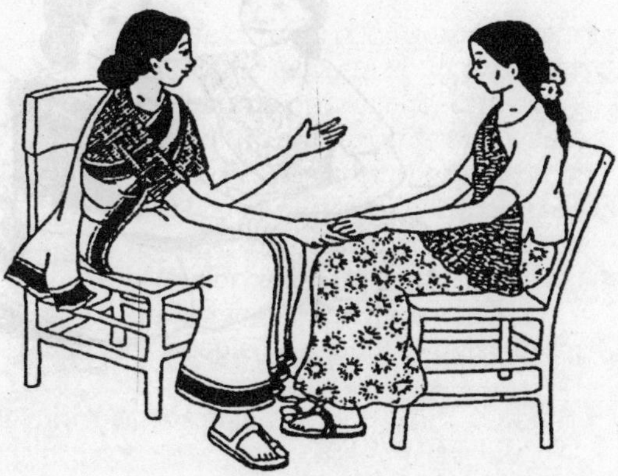

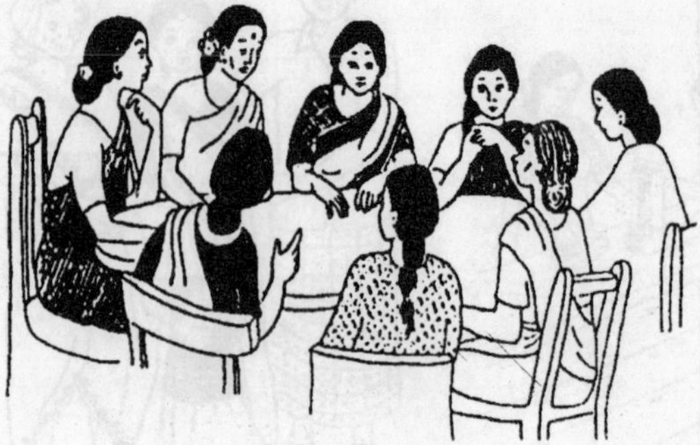

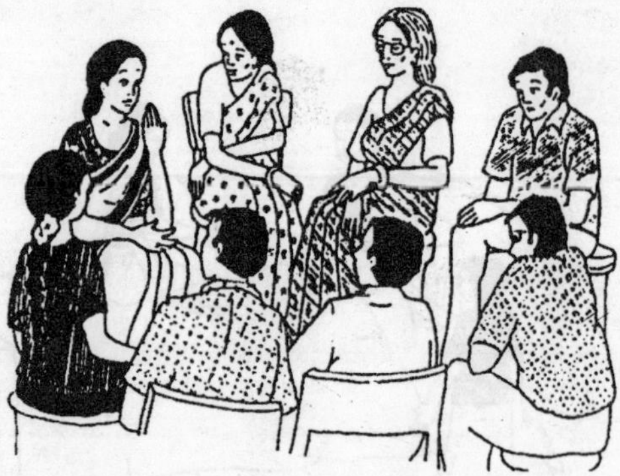

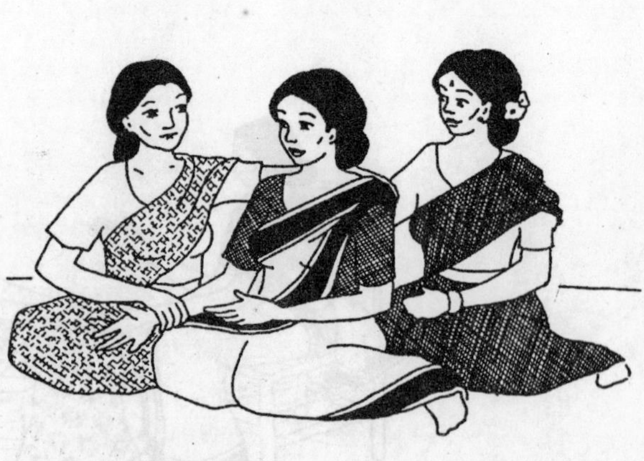

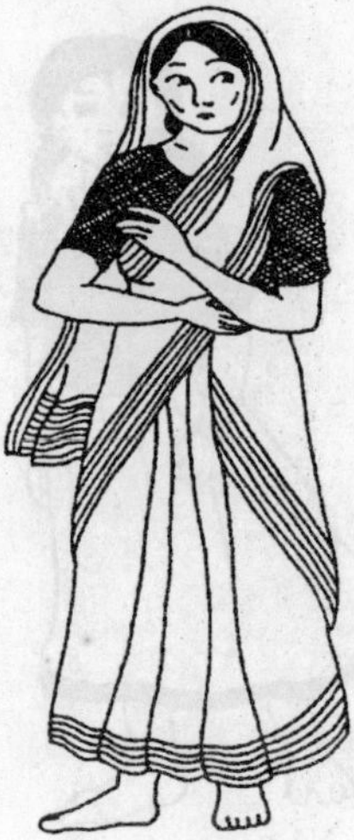

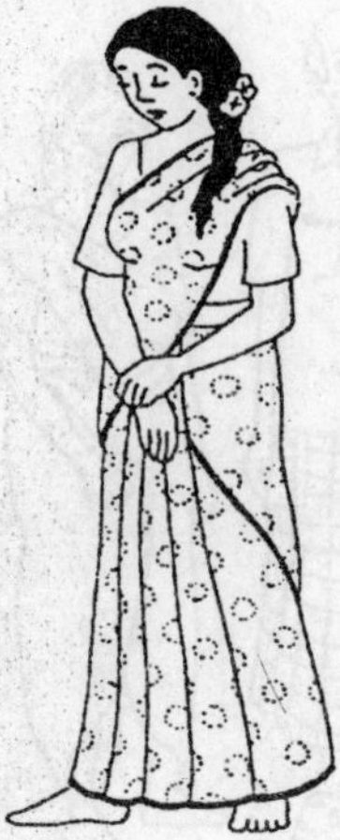

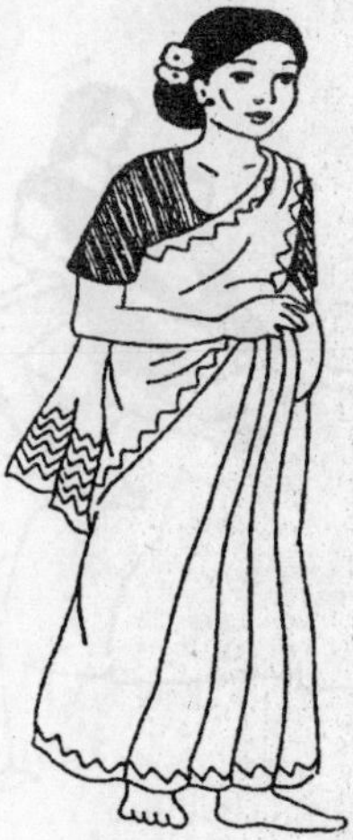

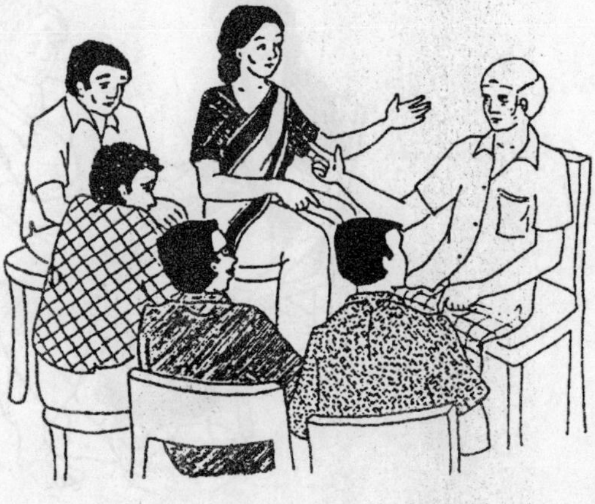

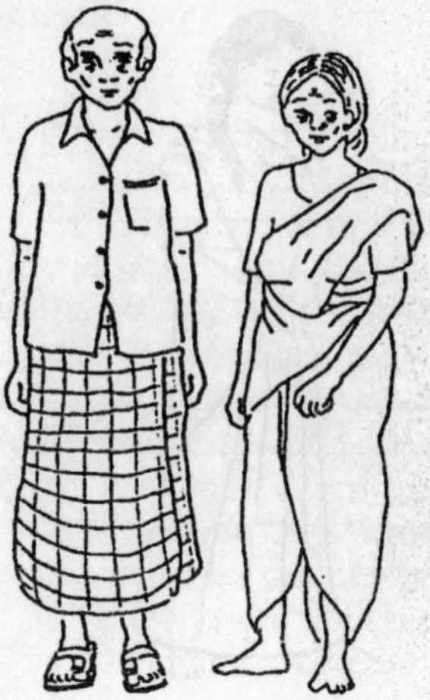

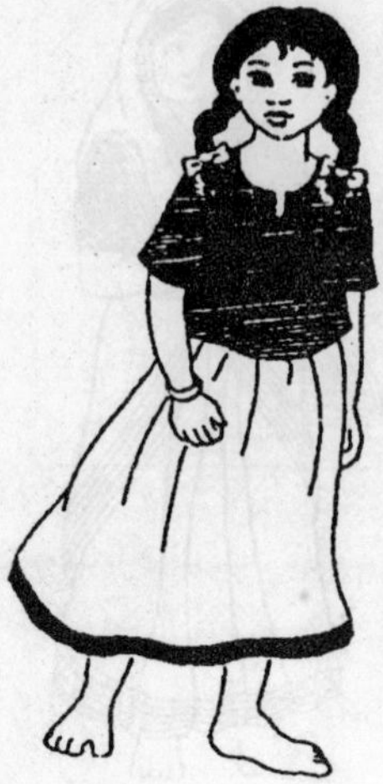

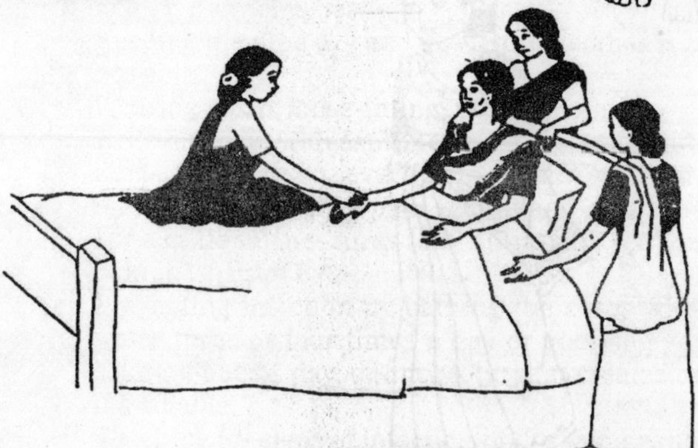

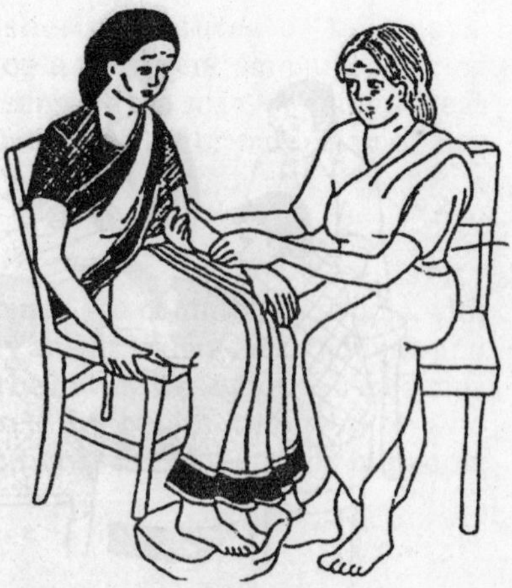

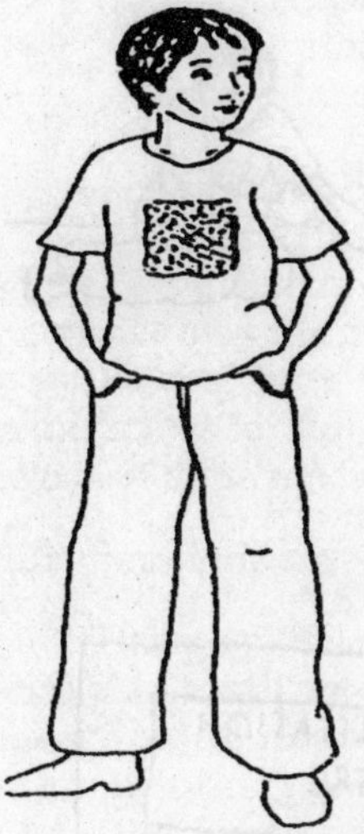

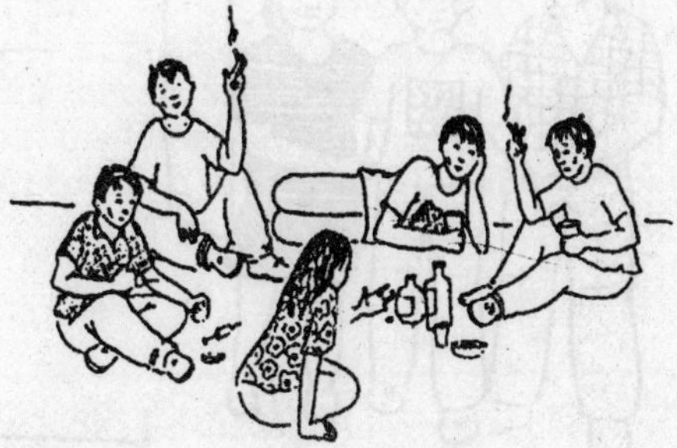

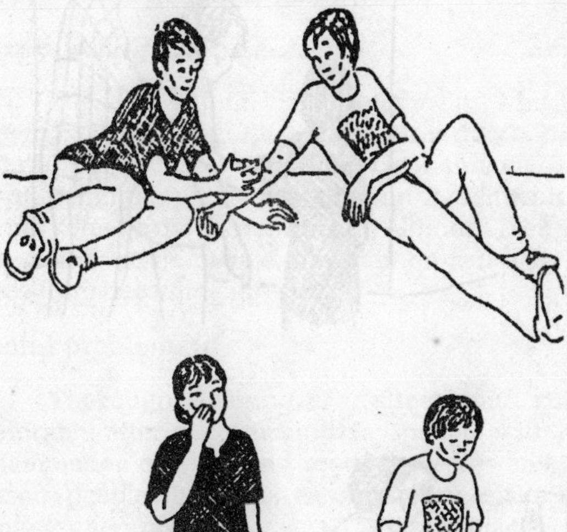

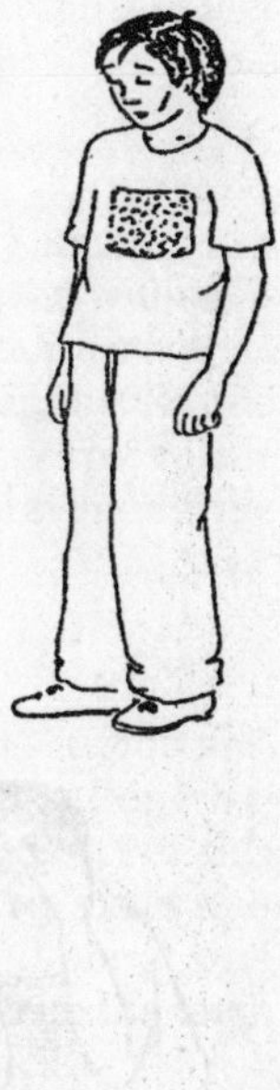

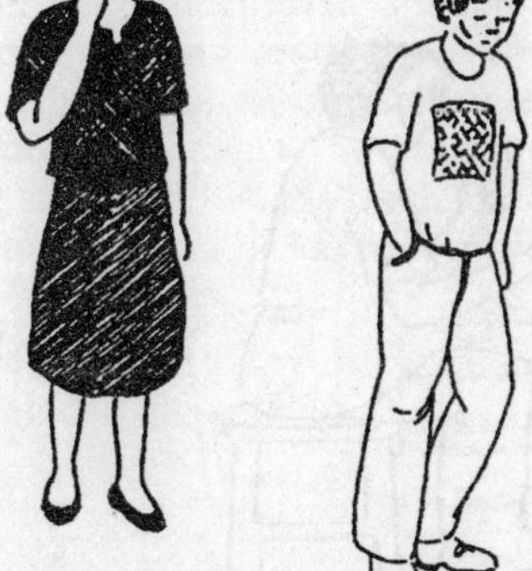

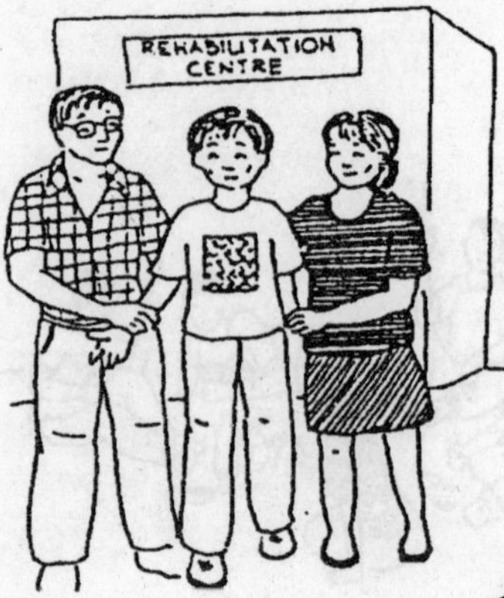
REHABILITATION
CENTRE

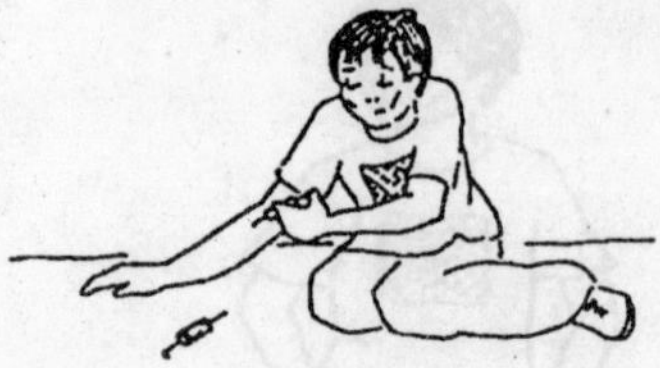

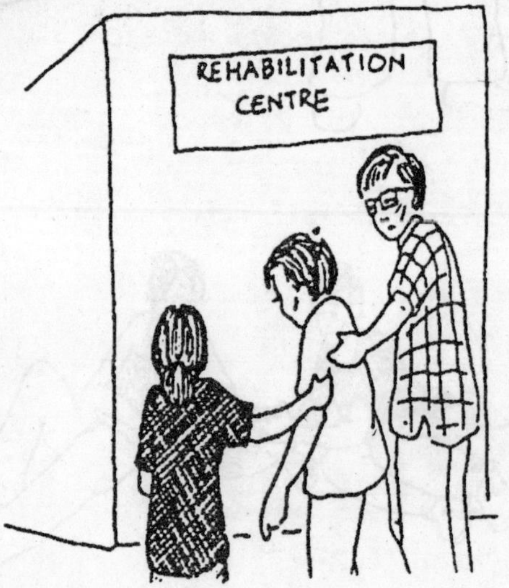
REHABILITATION
CENTRE

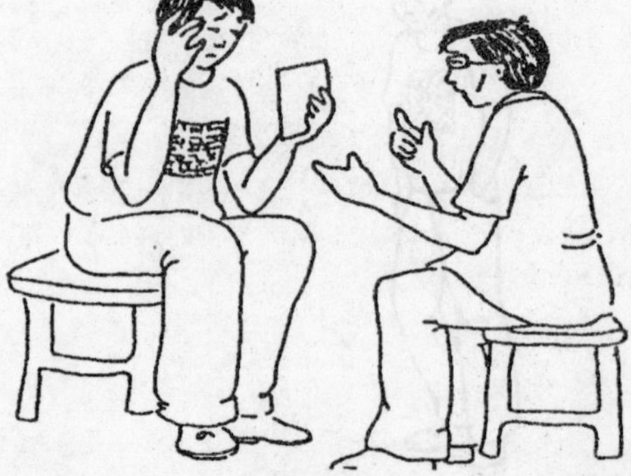

10

HIV/AIDS : A Pictorial Summary

AIDS IS A WORLDWIDE PROBLEM OF EXTRAORDINARY SCOPE AND UNPRECEDENTED URGENCY.

Estimated number of persons living with HIV/AIDS: 22.6 Million

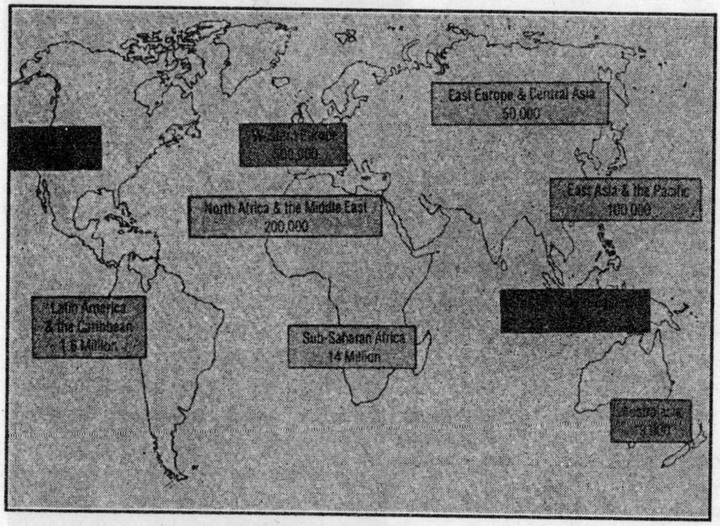

1,544,067 AIDS cases reported to WHO and UNAIDS from 164 Countries.*

Source: WHO, December 1996.

MODES OF TRANSMISSION

HIV/AIDS is transmitted in four ways:

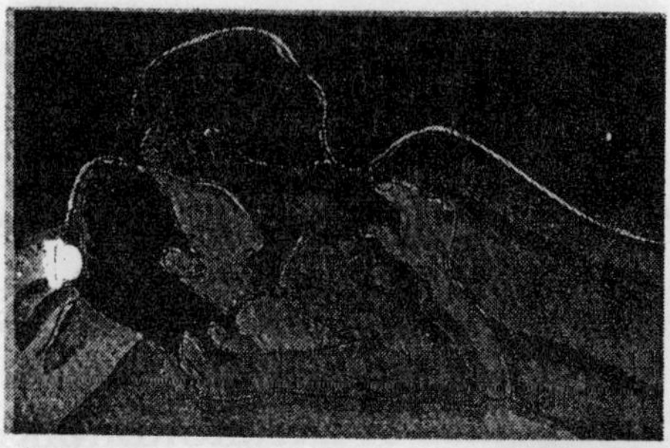

Sexual intercourse—from any HIV infected person to his or her partner (ı an to woman, woman to man, man to man). Women are more at risk than men.

Blood—through HIV infected blood transfusion or blood products.

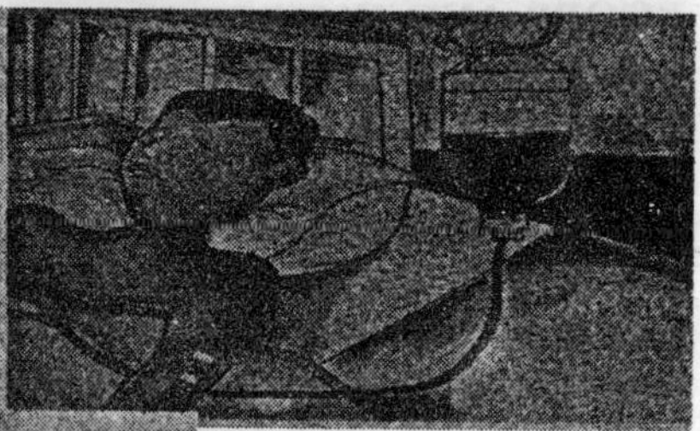

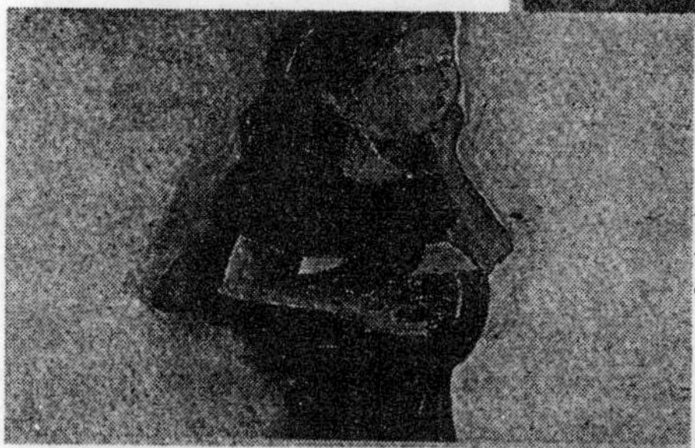

HIV infected mother to infant—before, during and after child birth.

Blood-sharing HIV contaminated needles or other skin piercing instruments.

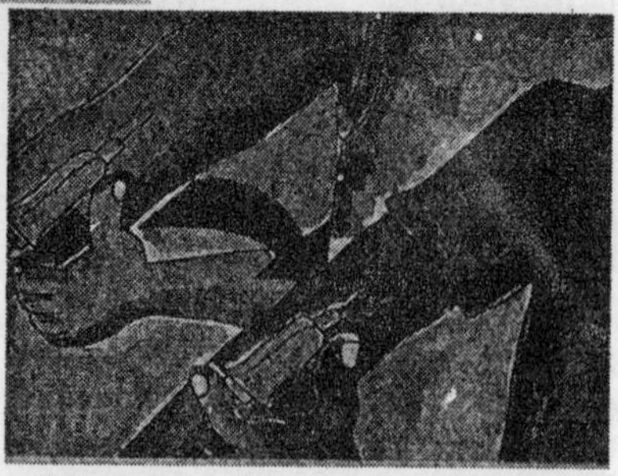

HIV Spreads through specific and Indentifiable Human Actions, All Subject to Human Influence and Control.

AIDS: WHO IS AT RISK?

What an individual "does" and not what he/she "is" determines the risk of infection.

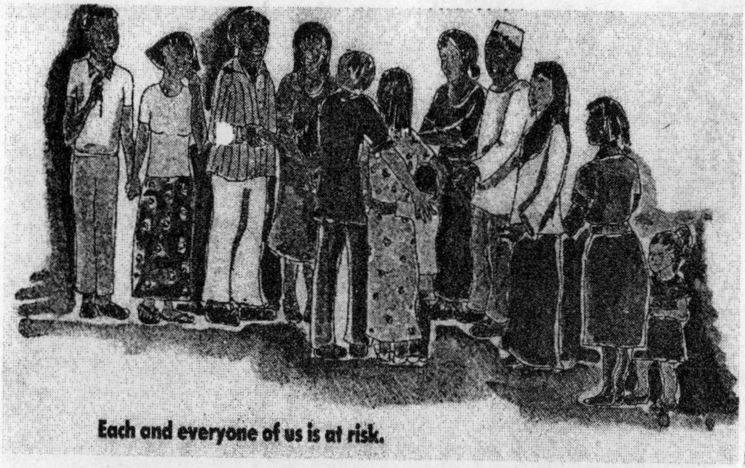

Each and everyone of us is at risk.

Certain behaviours carry particularly high risk of transmission:

- Those who have sex with multiple partners, especially when condoms are not used.
- Injecting drug users who share contaminated needles.

ADOLESCENTS AND YOUTH

During 1995, half of the newly infected in the world were adolescents and young adults.

Therefore, adolescents and young adults have the right to know about HIV/AIDS in order to protect themselves.

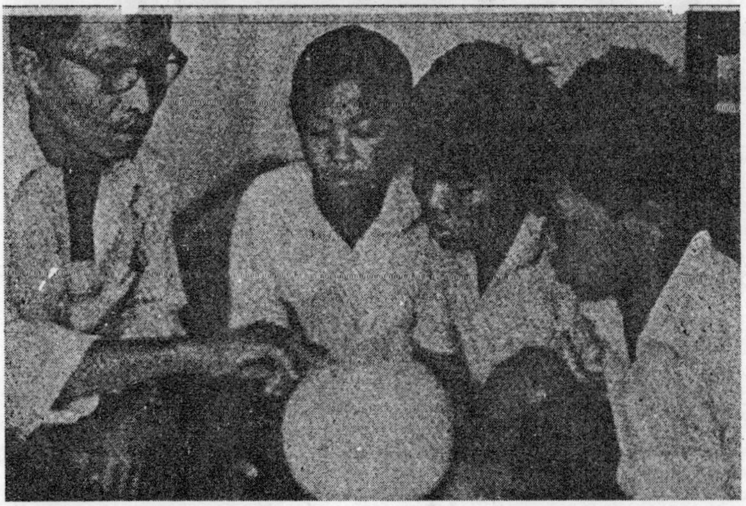

Sex education encourages a responsible attitude towards sex rather than early experimentation.

VULNERABILITY OF WOMEN

By end 1996, a cumulative total of over 2.8 million cases of AIDS will have occurred among women, or fifteen times as many as had occurred by the end of the 1980's.

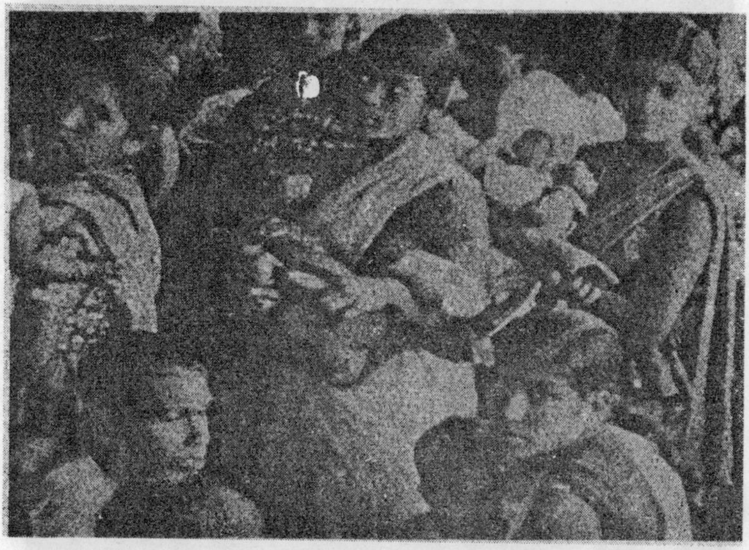

- Women are more at risk of getting the infection.
- The low status of women whithin the family and society further heightens their vulnerability.

Every woman must have access to information about HIV/ AIDS to protect herself and her family.

CHILDREN AND AIDS

Children are both infected and affected–a double tragedy

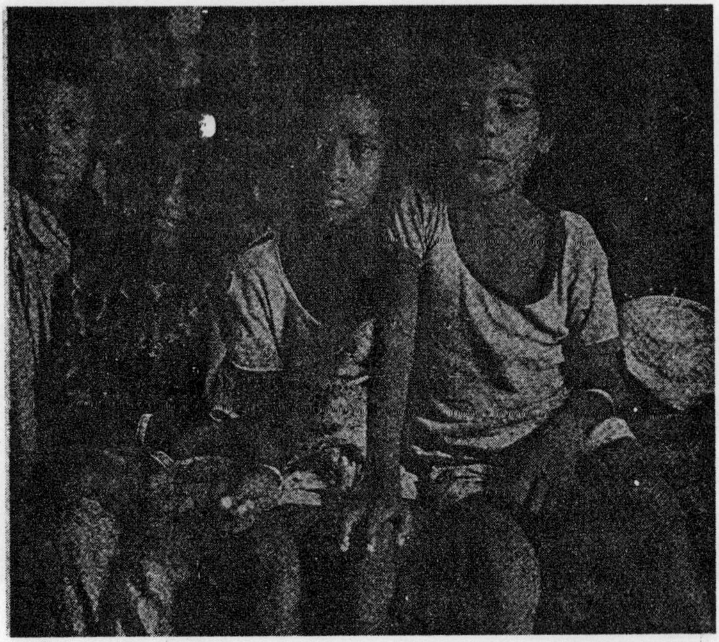

- As of December 1996, more than 2.6 million children worldwide were infected.
- If HIV continues to spread in the countries, there will be a great increase in deaths among infants and children.
- By the year 2000, 10 million children will be orphaned as their parents will die of AIDS.

Infants and children infected and affected by HIV infection/AIDS need special love and attention.

TUBERCULOSIS AND HIV–THE DEADLY DUO

Tuberculosis is the most common life threatening condition associated with HIV infection

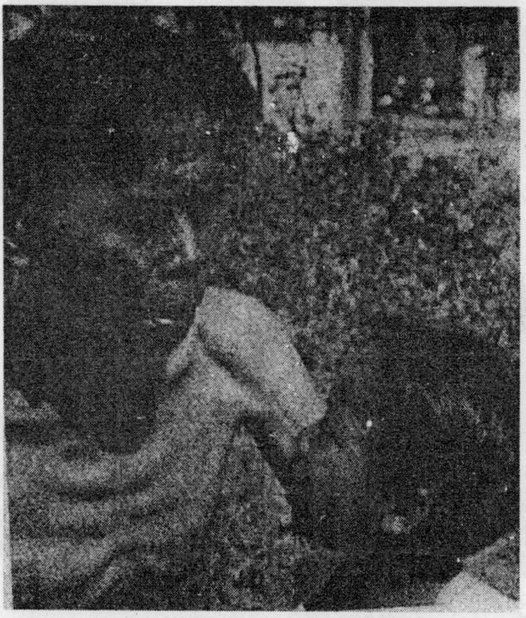

With the rise in HIV infection, Tuberculosis is also increasing as in Africa. The same is likely to happen in Asia as well.

HIV/AIDS IS NOT SPREAD THROUGH:

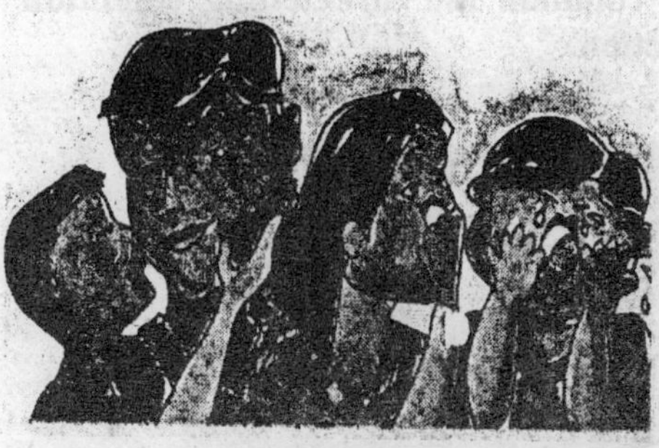

Touching or hugging, coughing or sneezing.

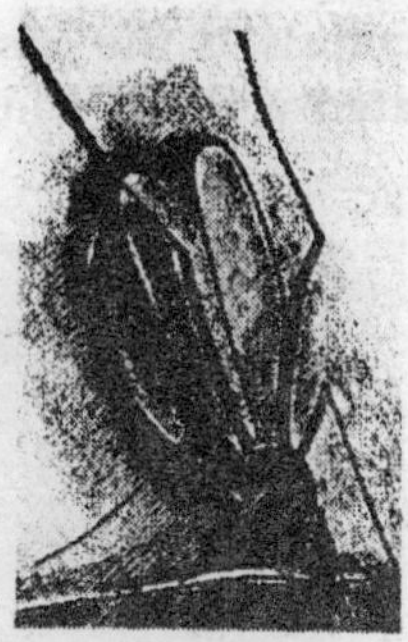

Mosquito & Insect bites.

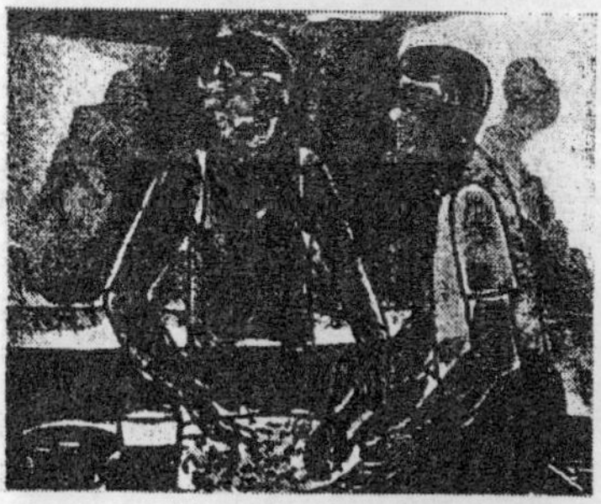

Water or food, glasses and plates.

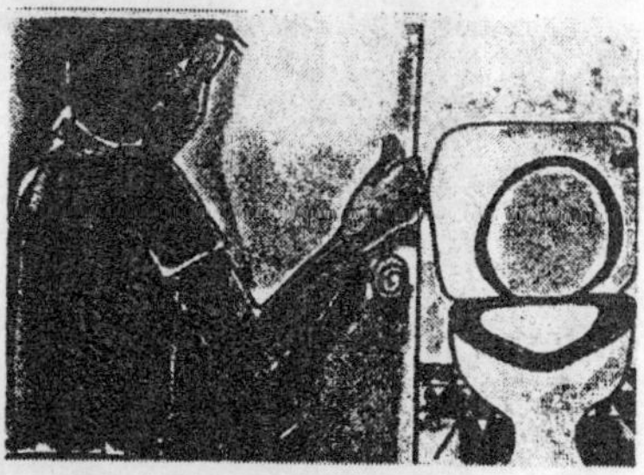

Toilets

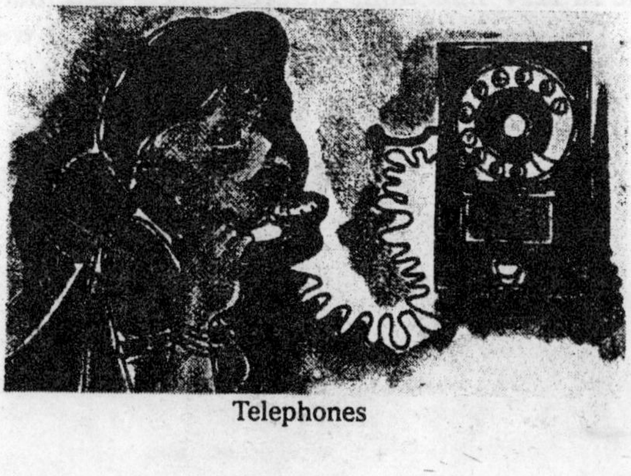

Telephones

AIDS is not spread through social contact with an HIV infected person or a person with AIDS or by Donating blood.

AIDS CAN BE PREVENTED BY:

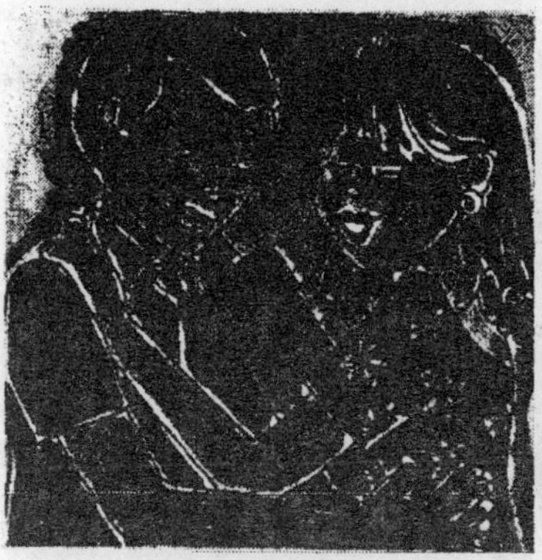

Being mutually faithful to your sexual partner.

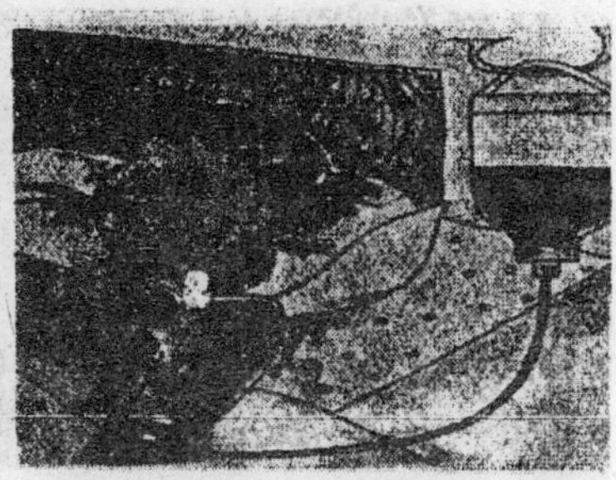

Using only HIV screened blood when required for transfusion.

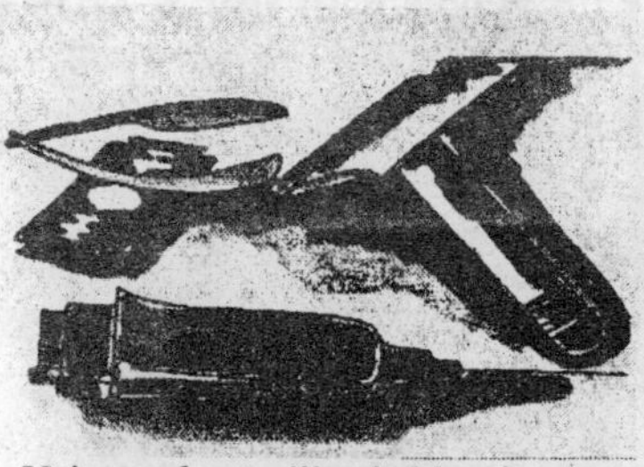

Using only sterilised skin piercing like needles, syringes, blades and razors.

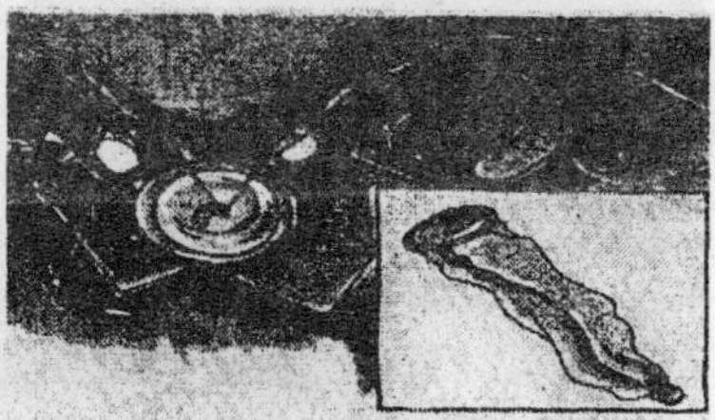

Using a condom for safer sex.

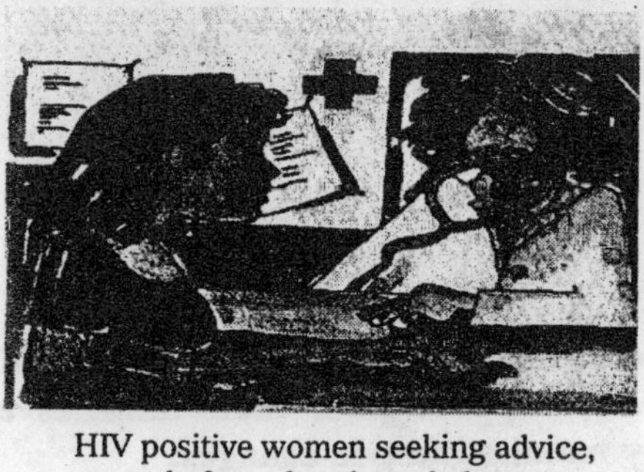

HIV positive women seeking advice, before planning a baby.

THE GLOBAL AIDS STRATEGY

- Prevent HIV infection
- Reduce the personal and social impact of HIV infection and AIDS.
- Mobilize and unify national and international

This calls for urgent action, commitment and solidarity.

AIDS: TIME TO ACT

- Fight denial, discrimination and complacency among governments, communities and individuals.
- Bridge the widening resource gap.
- Reduce the vulnerability of women.
- Provide young people with the knowledge and means to protect themselves.
- Set up strong prevention and education programmes.
- Ensure that humane care for people with HIV & AIDS is available everywhere.

CARE AND SUPPORT

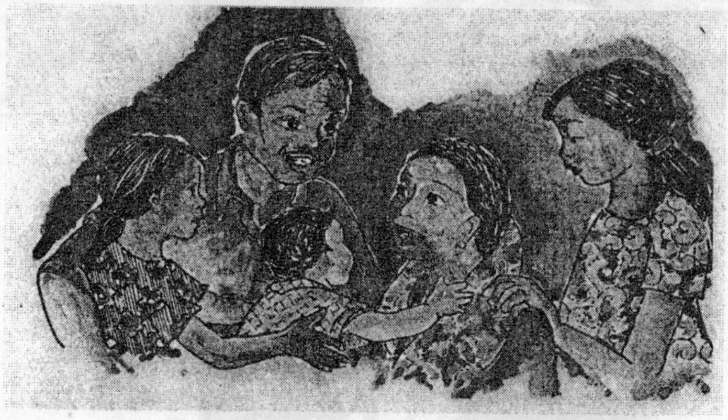

Living Positively

Persons infected with HIV can lead a happy and productivity life for years with support from their families and the community and by making lifestyle changes.

COUNSELLING

Helping people with HIV/AIDS to live positively

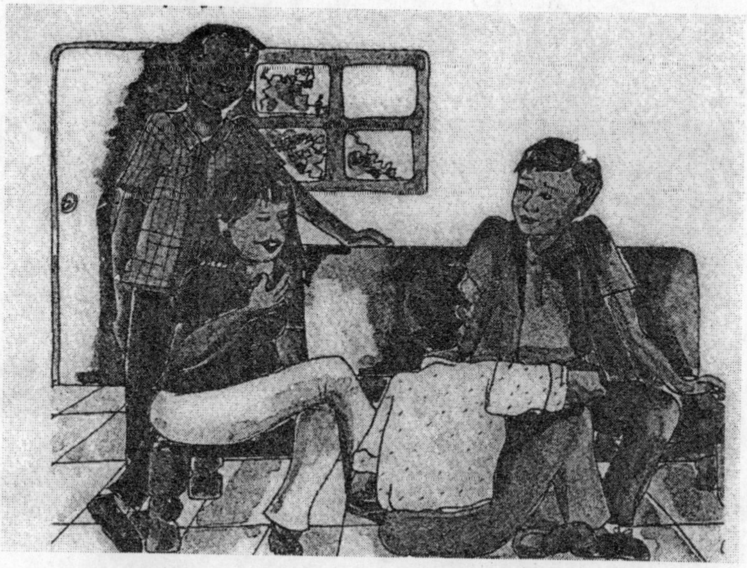

- To help those infected with HIV/Aids to live fully and productively
- To decrease stress related to HIV or high risk behariour
- To change high risk behaviour of those infected.
- To help families of HIV infected individuals and to support them to

Live Positively

AIDS IN THE SOUTH-EAST ASIA REGION IS SPREADING AT AN ALARMING RATE

There is no time for complacency

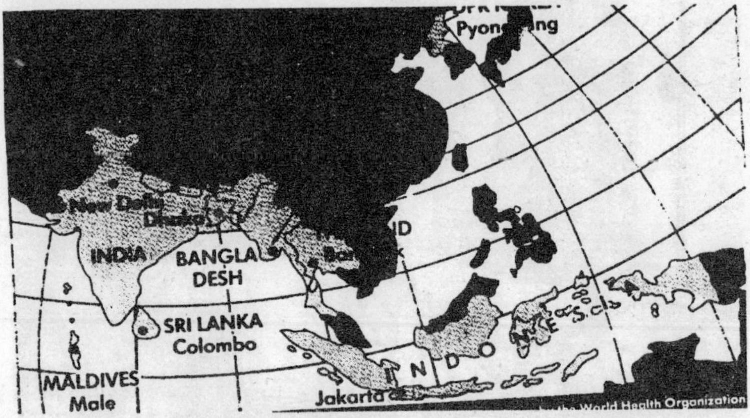

Currently estimated HIV infections	3.7 Million+*
Currently reported AIDS cases	49,000
Estimated AIDS cases in the Region by 2000	2 Million

Most of the estimated infections are in India, Thailand and Myanmar.

**December 1996*

AIDS PREVENTION AND CONTROL IN SOUTH-EAST ASIA

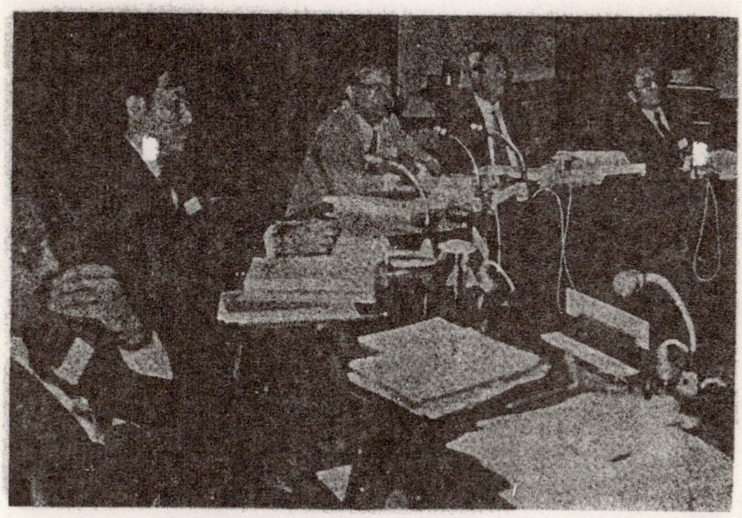

WHO provides support to national programmes for AIDS prevention and control in the following areas:

- Planning, implementation, monitoring and review of national response to the epidemic.
- Integrating AIDS prevention and care programmes into primary health care and promoting multi-sectoral response.
- Training and national capacity building, particularly in public health areas.
- Collaborating with UNAIDS and other co-sponsors.